THE LAW OF RESIDENTIAL HOMES
AND DAY-CARE ESTABLISHMENTS

AUSTRALIA AND NEW ZEALAND
The Law Book Company Ltd.
Sydney : Melbourne : Perth

CANADA AND U.S.A.
The Carswell Company Ltd.
Agincourt, Ontario

INDIA
N. M. Tripathi Private Ltd.
Bombay
and
Eastern Law House Private Ltd.
Calcutta and Delhi
M.P.P. House
Bangalore

ISRAEL
Steimatzky's Agency Ltd.
Jerusalem : Tel Aviv : Haifa

MALAYSIA : SINGAPORE : BRUNEI
Malayan Law Journal (Pte.) Ltd.
Singapore

PAKISTAN
Pakistan Law House
Karachi

The Law of Residential Homes
and
Day-Care Establishments

M. D. A. Freeman, LL.M.,

of Gray's Inn, Barrister
Reader in English Law, University College London

and

Christina M. Lyon, LL.B.,

Solicitor, Lecturer in Law, University of Manchester

LONDON
SWEET & MAXWELL
1984

Published in 1984 by
Sweet & Maxwell Limited of
11, New Fetter Lane, London
Computerset by Promenade Graphics Limited, Cheltenham
Printed in Great Britain by
Page Bros. (Norwich) Ltd.

British Library Cataloguing in Publication Data

Freeman, M.D.A.
    Law of residential homes and day-care
    establishments
    1. Institutional care—England—Law and
    legislation
    I. Title   II. Lyon, Christina M.
    344.204'3105   KD3299

    ISBN 0–421–25860–8

Preface

This book, we believe, fills a gap in the existing literature. It is the first book to cover comprehensively and, we hope, comprehensibly all the law relating to residential homes and day-care establishments. By including within one cover the law relating to children and young persons, the mentally disordered, the elderly, the sick and the handicapped we are providing virtually a social work legal textbook.

The law has undergone recent and radical transformation. Mental health law was reformed in 1982 (the new consolidating Mental Health Act 1983 came into operation together with new regulations on September 30, 1983). The Health and Social Services and Social Security Adjudications Act 1983 has made significant changes to child law as well as making an impact on most other areas of social services legislation. Both Acts are complex and require considerable interpretational skills. This book should enable the social worker to pick his or her way through the thickets of this new legislation.

In writing this book we have been assisted by any number of people. In particular we would like to thank Lorna Nix and Jacqueline Daniels of the Liverpool Social Services Training Staff, Chief Inspector K. Hoskisson of the Merseyside Police, and Barbara Wells, University College London's Law Librarian. The unenviable task of turning a messy manuscript into reasonable type was undertaken by the secretarial staff of Manchester University Law Faculty and particularly by Sandy McDonald of University College London. To them we express our indebtedness and thanks.

The law is stated as at August Bank Holiday weekend 1983, which we now hope to enjoy.

M. D. A. Freeman and Christina M. Lyon

August 1983

Contents

Table of Cases

Table of Statutes

Table of Statutory Instruments

Introduction

The general trend may be away from residential care and in favour of supporting those unable to care for themselves because of age, disability or other incapacity within the community. Nevertheless, a very large number of persons today are in children's homes, mental hospitals, nursing homes, old people's homes and other institutions.

This book aims to set out as succinctly as possible the very complicated legal frameworks which govern these institutions. It emphasises admission procedures, the rights of persons who live within the institutions, the duties and powers of social workers including residential staff and other personnel involved in the administration of the legislation. The book is comprehensive in its coverage. Within it is found most of the law which the social worker is likely to need in his or her daily routine.

The book is in three parts. Part I is concerned with the law relating to institutions concerned with the care of children and young persons. Part II covers the law governing the mentally disordered and the institutions provided for their care. Part III examines the law relating to nursing homes, mental nursing homes, old people's homes and other provision for the elderly, the chronically sick and the handicapped.

With increasing emphasis on care within the community, there is some account throughout of the powers and duties of social services authorities and other bodies to keep less privileged sections of the population within the community whenever possible by assistance of various kinds and other preventive work.

Part I
Children and Young Persons

1. Provision of Residential Accommodation for Children

I. *Children in the Care of the Local Authority*

(a) Historical outline

Provision for orphaned, abandoned or destitute children

The principle of localised provision of residential accommodation for abandoned, destitute or orphaned children has a history stretching back to the Elizabethan Poor Law. Originally housed together with able-bodied and the elderly in the general mixed workhouses, in the nineteenth century an increasing number of children were housed separately in district or barrack schools or later in the more attractive cottage homes. In addition, that century saw the burgeoning of homes provided by charitable benefactors or voluntary organisations, such as the Mary Carpenter homes for children of the streets and Dr. Barnardo's homes for boys, and such voluntary homes still feature in the residential child care system. By the early years of this century, and after much criticism of the local provision of residential care for children by people such as Mrs. Senior and Henrietta Barnett, the Poor Law Commission of 1905 recommended special homes for destitute and orphaned children, but the provision of residential care for such children remained haphazard and over the country as a whole, large numbers remained in workhouses (*Crowther*, 1981).

Although the Government in 1913 issued a directive that all children were forthwith to be removed from workhouses, it remained unfulfilled. The Poor Law Guardians were then directed to ensure

5

the removal of all children from the workhouses by 1915, but the war forced the repeal of that measure by the Local Government Board. After the war the Ministry of Health again issued orders that all children should be removed but these orders also ran into difficulties, partly from local boards who objected to the cost of provision of separate accommodation, and also because of problems with the building industry. The Ministry itself, however, seemed reluctant to enforce its orders, and a close examination of their reports issued in the 1920s reveals that many children were still being housed in the children's wards of general workhouses. Many of these children were there in order that they could be with their parents, who had no alternative but to seek relief from the workhouse.

Even by the late 1920s there was no coherent structure for the provision of residential care for orphaned, abandoned or destitute children. As with the Poor Law generally, it was subject to wide variations of local discretion, and to differing levels of local reliance on provision made by voluntary organisations. The pattern of varying residential provision continued up to 1948, using buildings which were or had been annexed to workhouses or district schools. Some authorities, however, had by this time established family group homes, much smaller units housing eight to twelve children, but all forms of accommodation were known generically as local authority children's homes.

In 1946 the provision of residential care for children came under the scrutiny of the Curtis Committee, whose report led to the establishment of Local Authority Children's Departments, and to the passing of the Children Act 1948 (*Curtis*, 1946). The Committee had been so appalled by the emphasis on deterrence practised in the homes, that they recommended a complete shift in attitude towards residential child care. Even in those children's homes where it had found that attempts had been made to adopt family models, the members noted a lack of attention to the needs of children as individuals; they had few toys or recreational activities, too much time was taken up with domestic chores for both staff and children and there was little contact with the outside world. The same was true whether the institution was a workhouse annexe, barrack school, cottage or family home. As a result of their investigations, the Committee was dubious as to the merits of trying to offer family life through extending residential care, and opted instead for positive moves to encourage placement of children with ordinary families. They were forced to recognise, however, the need to retain a residuum of children's residential homes, which they urged should be on a much smaller scale run on family group lines, aimed as near as possible at reproducing the actual conditions of family life. Admirable though this aim may have been, it inevitably produced strains on staff, who were expected to work long hours, often in cramped conditions with minimal assistance on the domestic side (*Davis*, 1981).

The Williams Committee Report in 1967 pointed out that the idea that residential care was just the same as the care of every family but on a larger scale resulted in the work of residential staff being seen as more or less the same sort of job as that done by any housewife with a fairly large family. Concerned to encourage the professionalism of residential workers within social work generally, the Committee was at pains to emphasise the enormous gap between the skills required by residential social workers and those needed in ordinary families. This was a gap which was to become even more apparent, when at the end of the 1960s, the Children and Young Persons Act 1969 resulted in the full integration of the resources available to meet the needs of children who were orphaned, abandoned, destitute or otherwise in need of care and protection, and those additionally who had found themselves in trouble with the courts.

Provision for children in need of control or protection

The basis for combining consideration of the provision for those two groups of children is actually historical. Concern about the causes of juvenile crime was very real by the beginning of the nineteenth century, and there was a feeling that juvenile delinquents might be drawn from particular social classes. To meet the problems of the actual delinquent and the potential delinquent, two schemes of residential care evolved: the reformatory to deal with the former, and the industrial school to deal with the latter (*Pinchbeck and Hewitt*, 1973). Into the class of potential delinquent, somewhat strangely, fell children in need of care and protection so that they too were admitted to Industrial Schools (*Eekelaar, Dingwall and Murray*, 1982). Although the distinction between the two types of schools was emphasised right up to 1896, Eekelaar *et al* report that the principle of deterrence could clearly be seen at work. Thus, the inmate children of industrial schools were perceived as being just as much at risk to society as at risk themselves. The underlying purpose of the reformatory was positive, involving the imposition of strict codes of discipline, whereas that of the industrial school was the promotion of the child's welfare by providing education and industrial training for the class of children from whom the inmates of reformatories were usually drawn. There had, however, been calls in the latter part of the nineteenth century for the assimilation of the two types of schools and in 1927 the Committee on Young Offenders again demanded their amalgamation stating that:

> "there is little or no difference in character and needs between the neglected and the delinquent child. It is often a mere accident whether he is brought before the court because he is wandering or beyond control or because he has committed some offence. Neglect leads to delinquency and delinquency is often the direct outcome of neglect."

Parliament adopted the report's recommendations and the Children and Young Persons Act 1933 abolished the differences between reformatory and industrial schools, which were amalgamated to form "approved schools." The legislative provisions under which children could be committed to these schools however were kept separate. Thus, children convicted of criminal offences were committed under section 57, and children characterised as in need of care and protection as a result of neglect or ill treatment by their parents, were committed to care under sections 61 and 62. Yet, though it was obvious that these groups might require very different forms of care, both groups ended up in approved schools. As members of the Ingleby Committee were later to comment in respect of proceedings under section 61, "these are not criminal proceedings, and so there is no lower age limit, and no finding of guilt yet the result may be what is regarded as the severest punishment for an offence namely, the sending of a child to an approved school."

While it might have appeared consistent to send children, who could be considered to be at risk of falling into bad ways because of their parents' neglect, it seems incredible that children who were the victims of their parents' ill-treatment could also find themselves in an approved school by virtue of section 61. The result therefore of the 1933 consolidating Act was that approved schools could end up as the home for delinquent, neglected and ill-treated children. Although the 1933 Act consolidated the reformatory and industrial schools into a single group, it did retain the pattern of central government management, regulation and inspection by the Home Office, which had developed in the 1860s. This had the inevitable consequence that approved schools were isolated from developments in other areas of residential child care, such as special schools and children's homes.

In the years leading up to the passage of the Children and Young Persons Act 1969 moves were made which broke down the barriers between the different forms of residential child care. After the Children Act 1948, all residential child care facilities were subject to the common administration and inspection powers of the Home Office Children's Department, which resulted in some cross-fertilisation of ideas. The influence of the local authority Children's Departments set up after the 1948 Act could clearly be seen at work in the approved schools in moves such as the building of house units in some schools to replace dormitories and common rooms, and the appointment of child care staff to the existing teams of trade training and teaching staff. As Cawson (1978) states "the increasing contact with social workers and the field services, the relaxation of regimes and lessening severity of sanctions in the schools reflected also the changing approach to delinquency in society as a whole during this period." She further comments that the 1969 legislation can therefore be seen as consolidating an emergent approach to the care of delinquent children, rather than creating a new one. The problem was that no *one* approach had emerged so that fifteen years later there is still an uneasy tension between the punitive and therapeutic approaches to the treatment of "delinquent" children. Large parts of the 1969 Act which emphasised the therapeutic approach remain unimplemented, and there has been a resurgence of faith in the efficacy of punishment, though backed up by little evidence of its success. The recent Criminal Justice Act 1982 underlines the popularity of this approach with the residential care order giving magistrates the power to insist that a child who is the subject of a care order should not live at home for a period of up to six months. (see below p. 52).

The 1969 Act completely altered the legal framework for the

care of children against whom there is a finding of guilt. It provided for the abolition of the former centrally controlled system of approved schools and their integration within the local authority system of children's homes. The provisions allowing juvenile court magistrates to commit children to approved schools for up to three years and to transfer parental rights to school managers were repealed. Under the Act, social workers were allowed to determine the nature of care for each child. Care could take the form of living in a community home with education on the premises (the term used for the old approved schools) usually after a period in an assessment centre; living in an ordinary community home provided by a local authority or voluntary organisation; or whilst on a supervision order undergoing residential intermediate treatment; or being allowed to be at home on "trial."

A further change aimed at underlining the switch from punitive to therapeutic approaches was the transfer in 1971 of the general responsibility for children's services from the Home Office to the DHSS, and the integration of these services with other local authority social services provision. Cawson states (1978) that the effect of all these changes was that the direct administrative links between the approved schools and the penal system were severed, and these schools were placed in the framework of provision for the care and treatment of those children in need. Thus, the potential existed as a result of the 1969 Act for children who had been committed into the care of the local authority to be placed in community homes with children in care under the 1948 Act (now the Child Care Act 1980). All children were therefore characterised as "in need" and if other accommodation or treatment was necessary, it was provided as part of the regional plan.

(b) The planning of accommodation for children in care

By whatever means a child comes into the care of a local authority in England and Wales, (see below p. 25) the Child Care Act 1980 lays down the ways in which the authority can discharge its *duty* to provide accommodation and maintenance for such a child. (s.21). Thus, the duty can be discharged by boarding the child out; (which is not the concern of this work, see *Hoggett*, 1981) by maintaining him in a community home, or any home which provides specialised facilities and services (s.80); or by maintaining the child in a voluntary home, the managers of which are willing to receive the child; or by making such other arrangements as seem appropriate to the local authority (s.21(1)(c)), which may include placing the child in a hostel or private children's home or allowing the child to be at home.

To enable local authorities more effectively and efficiently to plan and provide the various types of accommodation required, the 1969 Act introduced the idea of regional plans. Under those provisions, which were re-enacted in the Child Care Act 1980, s.31, each local authority in England and Wales was allocated by the Secretary of State for Social Services, to specific geographical areas of approximately five million people. In all there were some twelve regional planning committees established, each charged with the task of obtaining information about all the residential establishments and other provision for children in care within its region, and with assessing the overall requirements of the constituent authorities in respect of the accommodation of children and young persons in care. The membership of the Regional Planning Committee was governed by the provisions of the 1980 Act (Sched. 1) and after consideration of all the information compiled, each committee submitted to the Secretary of State, in accordance with their duty, a regional plan for the provision and maintenance of homes to be known as "community homes" for the accommodation and maintenance of children in care (s.31(1)). Community homes for which provision could be made by the plan included those run by local authorities or by voluntary organisations, where the local authority participated with the organisation in running the home. Homes provided by voluntary organisations were designated controlled or assisted depending on the degree of local authority participation.

In addition to indicating the homes to be included in the plan, the Committee had to put forward proposals regarding the nature and purpose of each community home included, and for the provision of facilities for the observation and assessment of children in care, and any additional necessary facilities. Resources could thus be used on a regional basis to provide a wide range of options for child care from residential nurseries for children under seven, through observation and assessment centres, community homes with education on the premises, and ordinary community homes, to special homes for physically handicapped children. The local authority also has the power to accommodate children in homes with special facilities, whose provision is directly controlled by the Secretary of State. Such provision is based on the idea that the particular facilities and services required for treatment are not likely to be readily available within community homes, and includes those units variously described as secure, special or intensive care units, and youth treatment centres (s.80). The Secretary of State further has the power to assist with the provision of secure accommodation within the community homes system other than in assisted community homes (s.81 and see below pp. 16–17).

By section 19 of the 1969 Act the regional plans were also supposed to contain the proposals in relation to intermediate treatment facilities to be made available for the use of children on supervision orders, subject to directions by the court. Under the terms of the supervision order, a supervisor and (following implementation of the Criminal Justice Act 1982) now the court also, may direct that a child reside for up to 90 days either in an ordinary community home or in one which offers certain specialised facilities (*DHSS*, 1972, 1983 and see below p. 82). There are those who think that regional plans should have been primarily directed towards these facilities in the first place rather than to the establishment of a system of residential and secure accommodation to deal with delinquent children. It is suggested and the point is perhaps well made that the requirement for up to 90 days treatment, not necessarily all in one period, might for instance have prevented a number of admissions for much longer periods in community homes with education on the premises (*DHSS*, 1977).

The extent to which each constituent authority had access to all these resources was laid down in the plan submitted to and approved by the Secretary of State (ss.32 and 33). Any changes or variations to the plan had to be referred back to him for his approval including proposals for changing the use of, or for opening or closing homes, though it seems some of these conditions were more honoured in the breach than in the observance. Thus, in *Attorney General* v. *Hammersmith and Fulham London Borough Council* (1979) the local authority proposed closing a particular children's home and an action was brought on behalf of one of the children in the home alleging that the closure was in breach of the authority's duty to give first consideration to the welfare of each child. The child's welfare, it was argued, was being jeopardised by the closure since the home had been the only stable factor in his life. The action failed, (a later one, *Liddle* v. *Sunderland Borough Council* (1982) did succeed) but the Court of Appeal ruled that the closure of a children's home amounted to a revision of the regional plan (s.35(*c*)) and the proposal should therefore have been submitted first to the Secretary of State for his approval. (See, further, *Freeman* [1984] J.S.W.L 44).

The Health and Social Services and Social Security Adjudications Act 1983, however, repealed the provisions of sections 31 – 34 of the Child Care Act 1980 and substituted a new section 31. Effectively this new section provides for the abolition of regional plans for the accommodation of children and for the transfer of responsibility to local authorities which can decide whether they wish to use their available resources jointly with one or more local authorities or on their own. In making such arrangements each local authority is under a duty to have regard to the need for ensuring the availability of accommodation of different descriptions and suitable for different purposes and the requirements of different descriptions of children. (C.C.A. 1980, s.31(2) as amended). Only time will tell what the practical effects of this change will be. Its most obvious immediate effect is the dissolution of the Regional Planning Committees, further evidence of the Government's dislike of what it sees as economically wasteful and unnecessary extra tiers in bureaucracy but like the Advisory Council on Child Care, also abolished by the 1983 Act, the loss of a body with general overseeing powers in a region may ultimately prove quite costly. The tasks formerly performed by the Regional Planning Committees will now have to be undertaken by each local authority, or by authorities acting together, resulting in a further drain on already scant local authority funds.

(c) Community homes

Definition

A community home, to be used by local authorities for fulfilling their functions under this section, is marginally better defined in the 1983 Act than it was in the 1980 Act. Thus, a community home may be either a house provided, managed, equipped and maintained by a local authority; or a home provided by a voluntary organisation, and depending on whether the local authority or the organisation is responsible for its management, designated as

either a "controlled" or "assisted" community home, Child Care
Act 1980, (s.31(3) as amended).

Community homes provided by voluntary organisations

The classification of community homes provided by voluntary
organisations under the 1983 Act into *controlled* or *assisted* affects
them chiefly as regards administrative measures, but may affect
them in other ways, for example in the ability to provide secure
accommodation (see below p. 17). The Secretary of State has quite
wide-ranging powers to provide for instruments of management
relating to the constitution of the management body of any voluntary home included in the plan, and the local authorities are given
certain powers. In the case of a *controlled* community home the
proportion of the body of management appointed by the local
authority must be two-thirds and in the case of an *assisted* community home, one-third. The remaining proportion of managers
representing the interests of the voluntary organisation are
appointed by that organisation in accordance with the terms of
their instrument of management (s.35, as amended). Should any
conflict arise between the terms of the homes trust deed and the
instrument of management, the instrument is to prevail over the
trust deed. The Secretary of State has the power after consulting
with the management body of a home and the relevant local authority to vary or revoke any of the provisions of the instrument of
management (s.36).

Management of a controlled community home. Where the home
is a *controlled* home, responsibility for the management, equipment and maintenance rests with the local authority designated in
the instrument of management, which exercises this function
through its managers. Thus anything done in relation to the home
is deemed to be done by the managers as agents for the authority,
and the managers are under a duty to keep proper accounts and to
submit them annually to the authority for its consideration. The
employment of staff at a *controlled* community home is under the
control of the local authority but the authority and voluntary
organisation can agree that a member of staff not appointed by the
local authority be employed to undertake duties at the home. Such
staff are then the employees of the voluntary organisation. (s.37).

Management of an assisted community home. Where homes are
designated as *assisted* community homes the voluntary organis-

ation is in charge of management, equipment and maintenance, and action taken by managers in relation to these homes is taken as agents of that organisation. The managers are also under a duty to keep proper accounts and records and to submit these annually to the responsible organisation. The employment of staff at an *assisted* home is generally a matter for the decision of the organisation, although the local authority is able to override any decisions as to hiring and firing made by the organisation (s.38).

Determination of disputes relating to controlled and assisted community homes. The 1980 Act re-enacts the provisions of the 1969 Act giving the Secretary of State power to determine disputes arising between local authorities and the voluntary organisation running *controlled* or *assisted* homes, relating to the placement of any child in such homes. The power possessed by the Secretary of State to determine disputes overrides any reservation of disputes to the authority or organisation provided for in the instrument of management. Upon determination of a dispute the Secretary of State can give such orders as he thinks fit to the local authority or voluntary organisation concerned. His powers extend to all disputes except those relating to religious instruction provided in the home, where the trust deed contains a term granting an ecclesiastical authority the power to decide any disputes (s.42).

Provisions relating to use as a controlled or assisted home. While a home provided by a voluntary organisation is used as a *controlled* or *assisted* community home, the provisions relating to registration of ordinary voluntary homes do not apply to them (see below, pp. 18–19).

Although the Secretary of State has powers to direct that any premises no longer be used as community homes (s.40 and see below, p. 17), it may be that voluntary organisations for one reason or another wish to discontinue running a *controlled* or *assisted* home. The statutory provisions are scarcely generous in either situation and indeed may constitute a strong disincentive to voluntary discontinuance when their implications are realised. Thus, the lengthy notice provisions and the heavy financial burdens imposed by the statute following a proposal to discontinue as a community home may result in the voluntary organisation having to transfer all or part of the premises or property owned by the home to the local authority (ss.43 and 44).

The Health and Social Services and Social Security Adjudications Act 1983 provides the local authority with the power to give notice to both the Secretary of State and the voluntary organisation concerned of its intention to withdraw their designation of the home as a *controlled* or *assisted* community home. The period of notice must be not less than two years, although where the body of managers give notice in writing that they are not prepared to continue as managers for that period, the Secretary of State can withdraw the instrument of management at an earlier date. Before making such an order the Secretary of State must consult both the local authority and the voluntary organisation, but if no such order is made the date upon which the home ceases to be controlled or assisted was that specified in the original notice. (C.C.A. 1980, s.43 as amended).

General provisions

All homes designated as community homes within the area of a particular local authority, or which elected to be included as such, are subject to any regulations as to their conduct as shall from time to time be made by the Secretary of State. The regulations which have been made make detailed provision as to the way in which the homes are run, particularly as this affects the children, and are considered in detail later (see below p. 63).

Provision of places of safety. Local authorities are directed by the statute to make provision in their own or in controlled community homes for the children who have been removed from a dangerous environment pursuant to a place of safety order (s.73). Where they find it impossible this provision within the local community home system and the child has to be accommodated elsewhere the authority has the power to defray any expenses incurred in looking after the child.

Provision of secure accommodation. Secure accommodation is defined by regulation 2 of the Secure Accommodation Regulations 1983 as accommodation in a community home for the purpose of restricting the liberty of a child resident therein. Accommodation cannot be so used unless it has first been approved by the Secretary of State, and in approving such accommodation the Secretary of State may impose such terms and conditions as he sees fit. Useful guidance for local authorities on how the Secretary of State would define restrictions of liberty for the purposes of the regulations is to be found in Annex B to the DHSS circular on the Secure Accommodation Regulations (*DHSS*, 1983).

Although it was originally thought that only a small minority of community homes would need secure provision, increasing use seems to be being made of this accommodation and deep concern was expressed in Parliament during debates on the Criminal Justice Act 1982. A report published in 1982 further revealed that the number of children being locked up had trebled in the previous ten years and that children as young as ten were being kept in secure accommodation (*Children's Legal Centre,* 1982). The Criminal Justice Act 1982 provided for the Secretary of State to issue regulations limiting which children can be placed in this type of accommodation, and the Secure Accommodation Regulations 1983 came into force on May 24, 1983 (see below, p. 67).

The extent of the availability of secure accommodation was indicated in the Children's Legal Centre report: thus by 1981 there were 558 secure places within the child care system, including two DHSS managed youth treatment centres (see *DHSS*, 1981), and 122 more were planned. An even greater demand for this type of accommodation by local authorities has arisen as the result of the directive limiting the issue of certificates of unruly character to boys aged fifteen and over which took effect in March 1982. Local authorities have since then been under an obligation to house in community homes all those boys aged 14–15 who might previously have been held in remand centres or prisons following the issue of a certificate of unruly character. A decrease in the use of secure places may however result from the tightening up of the conditions under which children may be kept in such accommodation by the Criminal Justice Act 1982 and the Secure Accommodation Regulation 1983 (see below pp. 67–8). Certainly, the Secretary of State has already indicated that the use of single rooms as secure places within ordinary community homes must cease by December 31, 1983 (*DHSS*, 1983 and see below p. 67).

Termination of use. The Secretary of State is given power by the statute to give directions that premises should no longer be used as community homes, be they provided by a local authority or by a voluntary organisation. Directions can be given where (1) the premises are unsuitable or (2) the conduct of the home is not in accordance with regulations made under section 39 (Community Homes Regulations 1972 and Secure Accommodation Regulations

1983) or (3) where conditions in the home are otherwise unsatisfactory.

(d) Voluntary homes

Apart from those voluntary homes provided by voluntary organisations included in the regional plan and designated *controlled* or *assisted* community homes, a good number of voluntary homes did not elect for inclusion and are thus outside the community homes system. They are referred to simply in the legislation as voluntary homes and are provided by such bodies as Dr. Barnardo's, National Children's Homes and the Church of England Children's Society. They are subject to different regulation from those designated as community homes, but it is always open to local authorities to make use of such homes where for example the home provides some specialised facility, or perhaps more commonly where the home is more accessible to parents and access visits will be facilitated.

Definition

A voluntary home is defined in the statute as any home or other institution for the boarding, care and maintenance of poor children, which is supported in whole or in part either by voluntary contribution or by endowments. It does not include a mental nursing home within the meaning of the Nursing Homes Act 1975 or a residential care home within the meaning of the Registered Homes Act 1984, s.1 (see below p. 218). The result of this definition is that if the voluntary homes receive not only poor children, but children who are also mentally handicapped, they will be subject to one set of provisions for registration and regulation in respect of the ordinary children, under the Child Care Act 1980 as amended, and to another set for the mentally handicapped under the Registered Homes Act 1984, s.22 (see below p. 218).

Registration

In order to function as a voluntary home, the home must apply to be registered in a register kept by the Secretary of State, the application to include the information prescribed by the Voluntary Homes (Registration) Regulations 1948. The decision to approve the application lies with the Secretary of State, who must if he refuses or if he grants approval subject to conditions, give notice in writing of his refusal, or of the conditions to the applicant (C.C.A. 1980, s.57 as inserted by H. & S.S. & S.S.A.A. 1983). A voluntary home can always have its registration cancelled by directions of the Secretary of State if it is not conducted in accordance with the Administration of Children's Homes Regulations 1951 (see below p. 70) or is otherwise unsatisfactory (C.C.A. 1980, s.57(4), as amended). The local authority as well as the home itself should be notified of the cancellation (C.C.A. 1980, s.57(7), as amended). There is, following cancellation, or refusal to give approval, or the attaching of conditions to an approval, provision to make representations to the Secretary of State within a period of fourteen days from receiving a notice in such terms (C.C.A. 1980, s.57B, as amended). Where this fails to achieve any change of mind on the part of the Secretary of State, then there is a right of appeal within 28 days of the service of notice of a decision to a Registered Homes Tribunal (C.C.A. 1980, s.57D as amended). On an appeal the Tribunal can confirm the Secretary of State's decision or direct that it shall not have effect, or vary any conditions which the Secretary of State may have attached to an approval, or direct that they cease to have effect (C.C.A. 1980, s.57D (4–5), as amended).

The Act further provides as did its predecessors, that those persons in charge of a voluntary home must notify the Secretary of State of certain particulars in respect of the home, in accordance with the Schedule to the Voluntary Homes (Return of Particulars) Regulations 1949 as amended by the Child Care Act 1980, s.59. These particulars include details about officials running the organisation by whom the home is provided, details about the children in the home, and the amount of any charges in respect of children in the care of the local authority being made to those local authorities. These details must be forwarded to the Secretary of State in respect of those homes established after the commencement of the 1980 Act within three months of their establishment, and thereafter in every subsequent year. For homes established prior to the Act particulars must be submitted in every year. Default in rendering particulars in accordance with these provisions renders the person in charge of the home guilty of an offence and liable on summary conviction to a fine (s.70).

(e) Private children's homes

As well as being able to use their own community homes, and those homes provided by voluntary organisations, local authorities may occasionally have to resort to placing a child in a private children's home, especially if these homes provide facilities not otherwise available. Although private homes were previously subject to little control apart from the general powers of inspection provided by the DHSS (see below p. 74) they are now subject to the Children's Homes Act 1982, as amended by the Health and Social Services and Social Security Adjudications Act 1983. In debates on the Act it was stated that about 175 homes are privately run for commercial purposes and about 2,500 children are looked after in these homes, placed there by about 50 local authorities (*H.C. Deb.*, 1982). Before placing a child in a private home a local authorities would be well advised to obtain information from the authority in whose area the home is as to the general standards of care exercised in the home and the level of any specialised facilities available to meet the problems of children with special needs. Private homes applying to be registered under the regulations which will be issued pursuant to the passing of the Children's Homes Act 1982, will be subject to similar requirements as those laid down for the registration of voluntary homes (see above, p. 18). Thus, the 1982 Act, as amended by the 1983 Act, provides for the same details to be submitted, and allows for the same conditions to be imposed on registration, for the annual review and cancellation of such registration, and for exactly the same system of representations and appeals relating to any decisions on registration (C.H.A. 1982, s.6 as amended). It is also provided that regulations will be made and it is likely that the 1951 Regulations may be extended to these homes, or that the new regulations will be almost identical in form to the earlier ones. Local authorities have now also been given powers to inspect premises in the same way as they can inspect voluntary homes (s.9).

(f) Provision of other accommodation

As well as its own community homes, homes provided by voluntary organisations or private bodies, a local authority may have to resort to using other types of accommodation. Some may indeed be under the control of the Director of Social Services for the area concerned, *e.g.* hostels for the mentally sub-normal (see below, p. 163, some may be under the control of the local education authority, *e.g.* special schools for handicapped pupils, and some may be under the control of the National Health Service, for example long-stay children's wards in hospitals, but in each case the authority is empowered to use any type of accommodation which may be suitable for the child's needs (s.21).

Special boarding schools for handicapped children do not come within the community home system, but as "schools" are subject to the investigative powers of local education authorities and the Department of Education and Science (see below, p. 76). The Warnock Committee Report reaffirmed faith in the system of special schools for physically handicapped children, and there is evidence that the provision of places in special schools is increasing (Statistics of Education 1961–1979). The provisions of the Education Act 1981 will no doubt give a further boost to their use in respect of children both over and under the age of five years (ss.1 and 2).

Where children in the care of the local authority are accommodated in the long-stay wards of hospitals, because they need prolonged medical treatment, they will be subject to the review powers of the local authority (see below, pp. 34–35). It is only where children in such hospitals are not there pursuant to action taken by the local authority that their position is relatively unregulated (see below, p. 77 and *Shearer*, 1980).

Local authorities are also empowered by the Child Care Act 1980 to provide financial assistance towards the expenses of accommodation, maintenance, education or training of young persons over 17, who have been in their care, but it has been argued that there is also a need for some form of unstaffed accommodation in which young people could live on a group basis, so that social workers could at least offer support and supervision during the critical last year or so of official care (*Leeding*, 1980). In some areas such accommodation is now being offered.

II. *Provision of Accommodation for Children not in Care of Local Authority*

Children who are not in the care of the local authority may nevertheless be placed in one of the forms of accommodation used by local authorities. It is still possible for children to be placed directly with voluntary organisations such as Dr Barnardo's and the Church of England Children's Society and such children may be housed in one of their voluntary homes or alternatively boarded out by them (see below, p. 56). Severely handicapped children may be assessed under the Education Act 1981 as being in need of special boarding school education, in which case they will be accommodated at one of the special schools recognised under the provisions of the 1981 Act, but they will not be in the care of the local authority and their parents retain rights over them (see below p. 58). Other children who are in need of prolonged medical attention may be looked after in the children's wards of long-stay hospitals but because they are not in care and not subject to any system of reviews may be forgotten (see below, p. 59).

III. *Forms of Residential Care for Children Provided in the Penal System*

Children over the age of 14 who are being held in, or who have been sentenced to a period of legal custody (see below, p. 59) may find themselves in all types of accommodation ranging from secure units in community homes, (see above, p. 16) through remand centres, young prisoners wings in prisons, detention centres and youth custody centres. Remand centres and prisons will usually house adults primarily but have wings or cells for young people, and are subject to the provisions of the Prison Act 1952 and regulations made thereunder including most recently the Prison (Amendment) Rules 1983.

(a) Detention centres

Detention centres are defined as "places in which male offenders not less than 14 but under 21 years of age are ordered to be detained for short periods under discipline suitable to persons of their age and description" (Prison Act 1952, s.43, as amended). The conduct of detention centres is governed by the Detention Centre Rules 1983 (see below p. 79) and are divided into junior and senior centres. Junior centres receive young persons under 17, and senior centres those in the range of 17 to 21. There are no detention centres for girls. A detention centre order can only be made when the court has been notified by the Secretary of State that a place in a centre is available, which is suitable for the convicted young offender. The committal areas for detention centres were revised in 1980 and more rigorous regimes have been introduced at four centres, including the junior one at Send and the senior one at New Hall, and a new senior centre has opened at Gringley Camp, Doncaster (*Home Office*, 1980). Following the implementation of the provisions of the Criminal Justice Act 1982 it was anticipated by the Home Office that there would be an increase in the number of young offenders being sent to detention centres by the courts albeit that the length of sentences has been reduced (see below, p. 59), (*Home Office*, 1983) and it is expected that some new centres will have to be built or existing ones expanded. (see below, p. 24).

(b) Youth Custody Centres

A youth custody centre is defined in section 43 of the Prison Act 1952 (as amended by the Criminal Justice Act 1982), as a place in which offenders not less than 15 but under 21 years of age may be detained and given training, instruction and work and prepared for their release. Before imposing a sentence of youth custody, the court should be satisfied that no other method of dealing with the offender is appropriate because it appears to the court that he is unable or unwilling to respond to non-custodial penalties or because a custodial sentence is necessary for the protection of the public or because the offence was so serious that a non-custodial sentence could not be justified (C.J.A. 1982, s.1(4)). To aid the court in reaching its decision a social inquiry report should have been prepared (C.J.A. 1982, s.2(2)). Whilst these criteria amplify the previous requirements of section 19(1) of the Powers of Criminal Courts Act 1973 which had to be satisfied before the imposition of a custodial sentence, it would appear that unlike the abolished sentence of Borstal training, no claims are being made for the rehabilitative qualities of youth custody (*McEwan*, 1983). The maximum youth custody sentence is the same as that which may be imposed on an adult, (s.7(1)) the minimum is generally four months, although in certain circumstances in the case of male offenders it may be less than four months but not less than 21 days (s.7(6)) unless imposed for breach of supervision on release where it may be less than 21 days (s.7(7)). Offenders serving sentences of 18 months or more will probably serve them in prison, unless aged under 16, when they should be sent to a youth custody or remand centre (s.17(2)). Girls of 15 and over may be sentenced to youth custody but it must be a sentence of four months or more in the case of girls aged 15 to 17 (s.7(6) and s.6(4)). There is thus no short sentence for girls under 17 comparable to that for boys (s.6(2)). Once over the age of 17 girls may well find themselves sharing the youth custody centres with older women, described as having a steadying effect (*House of Lords,* 1982) but who are in fact there because of the shortage of institutions for female offenders over the country as a whole (*House of Lords,* 1982). Indeed, the reason given for not providing a short sentence of youth custody for those aged 15 to 17 was that the number of girls who would get such short sentences would be too small to make it worth running an institution for them (*Young Offenders,* 1980 para. 2.4). The Government's evidence for this is that the last detention centre for girls, Moor Court, had many empty places but as McEwan points out (1983) Moor Court closed in 1969 and a startling increase in criminality in this age group has taken place since then. The provisions of the Criminal Justice Act 1982 relating to detention centres and youth custody centres serve to emphasise the Government's faith in the "short sharp shock" treatment (see further below, pp. 59–60). Indeed on the publication of the original proposals forming the basis of the new sentence, the Government admitted that they represented its firm commitment to custodial provision for some juveniles, which ran directly contrary to section 7(3) Children and Young Persons Act 1969, under which detention centres were to have been phased out (*Home Office, Welsh Office,* 1980).

2. Routes into Residential Care and their Consequences

General

The means by which and the bases upon which a decision is reached that a child be placed in the care of a local authority, or that parental rights may be assumed in respect of him, have been discussed elsewhere in this series. An attempt has been made to avoid unnecessary overlap but some must inevitably occur if a clear picture of the legal provisions affecting children in residential care is to emerge. Wherever fuller discussion of various issues is deemed desirable, reference should be made to these companion volumes (*Hoggett*, 1981 and *Smith*, 1979).

The position of children placed in the residential care of the local authority voluntarily or following civil or criminal proceedings is first considered; next, the position of children placed in voluntary or private children's homes; then the somewhat anomalous position of children in special schools and long-stay hospitals; and finally, the position of children in penal residential establishments pursuant to criminal proceedings. In each case the rights, powers and duties of the caring body, and parents and the children is examined. By way of conclusion the position regarding legal responsibility for the acts of children in care or legal custody is considered.

I. *Children in Residential Care following Voluntary Action, Civil or Criminal Proceedings*

1. Reception into Care under Child Care Act 1980, s.2

A large number of children in the care of local authorities in

England and Wales are in care as a result of a voluntary arrangement between the local authority and the parents or guardians. No statutory court order is made and the local authority does not possess full parental rights. During the year ending March 1980, 70 per cent. of the children admitted into care in English and Welsh local authorities were admitted on a voluntary basis, the chief reason for admission being the inability of the parents to provide care, or desertion by a parent (*DHSS*, 1982).

The Child Care Act 1980 (henceforth the 1980 Act) places the local authority under a duty to receive into its care any child appearing to them to be under the age of seventeen who, *either* (a) has neither parent nor guardian or who has been and remains abandoned by his parents or guardian or is lost, *or* (b) whose parents or guardian are for the time being or permanently prevented by reasons of bodily disease or infirmity or other incapacity *or any other circumstances* from providing for him proper accommodation, maintenance and upbringing. In each case the intervention of the local authority must be necessary in the interests of the child's welfare (s.2). The initial responsibility for receiving a child falls on the local authority in whose area he is, but a transfer of responsibility can occur at a later time to the authority in whose area he normally resides.

The decision to intervene is entirely a matter for the local authority, and will not be reviewed by a court provided it acted with propriety (*Re M*, 1961). The wording clearly however envisages some discretion; thus how it discharges its duty and which cases are given priority is a decision for the social services department. Care under this section is voluntary and no power is given to the authority to force a parent to place his child in care, a point stressed in debates on the 1948 Act and reiterated by Lord Scarman in the recent case of *Lewisham London Borough Council* v. *Lewisham Juvenile Court Justices* (1979). The provision empowers local authorities to receive a child without parental consent where the child is abandoned, lost or where the parent's incapacity is such that he cannot express his consent (s.2(1)(*a*) and (*b*)). If the authority does wish to take the child away against the wishes of its parents some other procedure must be utilised, for example, seeking a place of safety order under the Children and Young Persons Act 1969, s.28 (see below, p. 48).

Many local authorities adopt the practice of obtaining the written consent, wherever possible, of parents before receiving children into their care, but this is not required by law. There are DHSS leaflets available for use by local authorities which give vital information to parents whose children have been received into care, and which also request details from the parents about their children. (*DHSS*, 1977, and see *Bevan and Parry*, 1979). Most, if not all, of the information given by parents about their children should be passed on to the residential workers, so that they have the fullest picture of the child in their care.

Although the initial reception into care may be on a *voluntary* basis, as Lord Scarman has commented "this is a not wholly accurate term but in common use" (in the *Lewisham* decision, see above, p. 26), section 2 places the local authority under a duty not only to receive a child but also to keep the child so long as his welfare requires it, and he is under 19 (s.2(2)). Thus, while the child remains in care, a shift occurs in the location of rights, powers and duties in respect of that child, with the balance perhaps tipped in favour of the local authority. The provision does *not* however authorise the keeping of the child if any parent or guardian desires to take over the care of the child, and furthermore it places a duty on local authorities to endeavour to secure that the care of the child is taken over by a parent or guardian or relative or friend wherever it appears to them consistent with the welfare of the child so to do (s.2(3)). The drafting of the whole of section 2 is awkward and the relationship between subsections (2) and (3) difficult if not impossible for local authorities to administer (*Lyon*, 1979, *Freeman*, 1982).

Most of the other provisions relating to children received into care are less problematic and many also apply to children who are the subject of 1969 Act care orders, however made, and to children committed to the care of the local authority in other proceedings (see below, pp. 43–47). When discussing the position of these other children reference will therefore be made back to the relevant portions of this section to avoid duplication.

Consequences

Under the section 2 procedure, the local authority does not acquire the status of a parent and simply has physical possession of the child, subject to the provisions of the 1980 Act (*Freeman*, 1982; *cf. Maidment*, 1981). The Act imposes certain duties upon the authority such as the promotion of the child's welfare throughout his childhood (s.18), the provision of accommodation and maintenance (s.21) and the obligation to review the child's progress in care (s.20) but no parental rights as such are bestowed.

The position with regard to parental rights of access to children in voluntary care does seem to have been clarified by the enactment of new sections 12A–G of the Child Care Act 1980. The new provisions were inserted by section 6 and Schedule 1 of the Health and Social Security Services and Social Security Adjudications Act 1983, and introduce a new appeals procedure for parents whose rights of access to their children in care are *terminated* by the local authority. The new appeals structure introduced by the 1983 Act applies to any child in the care of a local authority in consequence of: a care order including an interim order under the Children and Young Persons Act 1969; a committal order under section 23(1) of the same act; orders committing the child to the care of the local authority under section 2(1) of the Matrimonial Proceedings (Magistrates' Courts Act 1960, section 10(1) of the Domestic Proceedings and Magistrates Courts Act 1978, section 2(2)(b) of the Guardianship Act 1973, section 17(1)(b) of the Children Act 1975, section 26(1)(b) of the Adoption Act 1976 and section 36(2) or (3)(a) of the Children Act 1975 and finally a resolution under section 3 of the Child Care Act 1980. The new procedure specifically does *not* apply to a child in the care of a local authority in consequence of an order made by the High Court or to children who are simply in care under the Child Care Act 1980, s.2 and in respect of whom no parental rights resolution has been passed (C.C.A. 1980, s.12A). Prior to the passage of the new provisions it was accepted by the DHSS, local authorities and the judiciary that in practice local authorities generally controlled access arrangements to children in "voluntary" care by their parents, although a number of commentators had argued that the legal position was far from clear (*Thomson*, 1975; *Maidment*, 1981; *Freeman*, 1981). The view of the former group was that as a matter of practice to allow otherwise would be to wreak havoc in the administration of the local authorities' duties under the various Children Acts (Ormrod L.J. obiter in *Re Y*, 1975), while that of the latter was that access was far too important a right in parent and child to be waived by administrative action without any right of appeal. From the wording of the new provisions, it would seem that it is implicitly accepted by the legislature that local authorities do have the unchallengeable power in relation to children in their care specifically covered by the new provisions (see above) to make arrangements for, and restrict access by, parents, though their rights to terminate such access altogether have now been expressly subjected to judicial review. Thus, section 12A(4) of the Child Care Act 1980 states that "a local authority are not to be taken to terminate access for the purpose of these provisions where they propose to substitute new arrangements for access for existing arrangements." The statute clearly acknowledges the local authority's rights to control such arrangements though *not* in relation to children only in voluntary care and thus to restrict parents' rights and moreover specifically excludes any challenge to the local authority's powers in this respect in the courts. This approach confirms the judicial view referred to earlier *except* in relation to children in voluntary care and seems to coincide with that of Lowe and White (1979) who have argued that "from the practical point of view it is essential for the authority to be able to limit access in so far as it is in the long term interests of the child since the parent could otherwise thwart attempts to provide consistent and proper care for the child."

To omit children in voluntary care from the protective ambit of section 12A indicates that the right of parents to have access to such children cannot in law be terminated by the local authority, or even be controlled in the same way as for those children specifically covered by the new provisions (see above). It is to be hoped in any event that the circumstances would never arise under which a local authority would attempt termination since section 2 care was only ever intended to be temporary care provision, and if more permanent arrangements are deemed necessary for the child, steps should first be taken to assume parental rights rather than be forced into such action by a premature move to terminate access. In any event if such a move to terminate access is made by the local authority in relation to a child in voluntary care and the parent objects, or indeed where the local authority is proposing to change existing arrangements, then where the child has been in care for less than six months the parents can remove him immediately, or where he has been in care for more than six months, give notice of intention to remove him (see below, p. 32). The giving of such notice may either prompt the local authority to reconsider any moves to terminate or restrict access, or to take action to pass a parental rights resolution (see below, p. 35). Where such a resolution is passed the child then comes within the provisions of section 12A–G and the parent can appeal any notice proposing to terminate his right of access.

Nevertheless one of the main reasons influencing a social services department's decision to place a child in a children's home rather than with foster parents may often be that access is facilitated, and the work towards rehabilitation of the child with its natural family, envisaged by section 2(3), rendered much easier. Indeed, one recent study (*Aldgate*, 1977) has demonstrated that parents are more inclined to visit children who are in such homes than those who are with foster parents, and ultimately this must materially affect prospects for rehabilitation. In order to improve these prospects, local authorities do have the power to defray the expenses of parents in visiting their children where hardship would otherwise arise (s.26). Although local authorities do have the power to control access and much of the responsibility for organising access will devolve on residential staff, Aldgate's study revealed that parents felt that the children's homes provided much greater flexibility over foster homes in arranging access which fitted in with their own domestic arrangements. This was particularly the case for parents who were in full-time employment.

Where parents fail to keep access appointments, residential staff should be aware of the potential importance for future decision-making about the child, of keeping an accurate record of such failures. A pattern of failure over a period of time could provide a basis for the subsequent passing of a parental rights resolution, and at a much later date as supportive evidence for the dispensing of parental agreement to an adoption on the grounds of persistent failure to discharge the obligations of a parent (s.12(2)(c) of the Children Act 1975). The responsibility for maintaining contact with the local authority and informing it of their whereabouts, so that access visits can be arranged, lies with the parents (s.9(1)). (But see *Family Rights Group*, 1983). Failure to inform the local authority of their whereabouts for a period in excess of 12 months can lead to the parents being deemed to have abandoned the child, which is a ground for the assumption of parental rights (s.3).

Removal of child from care of local authority

Although the length of time which the child spends in care does not of itself affect the local authority's legal status it may affect the parents' power/right to reclaim the child from that authority. "Parent," for the purposes of the statute, is defined as any person with a *legal* right to the child, normally both parents of a legitimate child, the mother of an illegitimate child or any guardian however appointed (s.2(6)). Thus, for example, where in divorce proceedings a court has given custody to the mother who later places the child in care, the father is not entitled to discharge the child from care unless the local authority agrees, and if it refuses his only course of action would be to return to the divorce court and to ask for an order varying custody. (*E. v. E. and Cheshire County Council (Intervener)*, 1979).

Problems may arise and the local authority be placed in a position of many conflicting duties (see s.2(2), s.2(3) and s.18) when a parent demands his child's return and the local authority does not think that a return at that time, or perhaps ever, would be beneficial for the child. Can the local authority in these circumstances refuse to hand over the child? The position where the child has been in care for *less* than six months is still far from clear, that where the child has been in care for longer than six months more so following the decision in the *Lewisham* case (see above). Needless to say, the actual physical problem of what to do with the child and how to deal with the parent in such situations, will in many cases in the first instance fall on the residential social worker, and none of the judges in the *Lewisham* case satisfactorily dealt with this practical predicament.

Child in care for less than six months. Where a parent demands the immediate return of a child who has been in care for less than six months, the child according to the *Lewisham* decision, remains in care until the parent collects the child. The parental request does not terminate care; it is a signal for action to be taken by the local authority (*Lyon*, 1979). As long as the child physically remains in the care of the local authority it can take further legal steps such as passing a section 3 resolution, if grounds exist, or the taking out of a wardship summons. Certainly, if the local authority is legally to justify refusing to return the child in accordance with section 2(3), some such action must be taken. Where a child has been in care though for less than six months, and there is real concern at the prospect of the child being prematurely reclaimed, preventive action in the form of a parental rights resolution or wardship should have been considered at an earlier stage, rather than running the risk of hastily taken proceedings failing. Given that a parent may well turn up at the children's home and purport to give the authority notice by informing the residential staff of his decision, it is important that they too should know the emergency procedures to be followed in such circumstances.

Child in care for six months. If the child has been in care for six months, the parent must give the local authority 28 days' notice "in writing" of his intention to remove the child (H. & S.S. & S.S.A.A. 1983, Sched. 2, para. 48(*a*)). The authority, therefore, has an extra 28 days "breathing space" in which to take such action as may be required to protect the interests of the child, though this was not primarily the reason for the enactment of the provision. The principal reason for the 28 days period was to enable the local authority to take time to prepare the child, and to give such assistance as may be necessary to parents, so as to enable the transition from the children's home back to the parents to proceed more smoothly. The imposition of a transitional period after the child had been in care for more than six months was in recognition of the fact that after that time the prospects of the child's returning home successfully diminish quickly (*Rowe and Lambert*, 1973) and long-term measures such as the assumption of parental rights might be more appropriate at that stage. Where a decision has already been reached that a child should not return home, the local authority should not wait to take action until the parent makes a move. This could arouse suspicion as to the motives for such reaction, little or no preparation work with parents or children will have been done, and feelings can tend to run quite high.

Custodial rights. Whilst the child remains in the care of the local authority under section 2, the authority does have physical custody of the child and the responsibilities which go with that. In addition to the duties of promoting the child's welfare (s.18) and providing him with accommodation and maintenance, however, the statute also empowers the authority if necessary in the interests of the public, to disregard the duty to promote the child's welfare and act in such manner as it thinks fit (s.18(3)). This may include, for example, the power to restrict the child's liberty by placing him in secure accommodation subject to the rights of appeal to the court laid down in the Child Care Act 1980, s.21A (see below). The Secretary of State is also able to give directions under the statute to a local authority with respect to a child in its care, for the purposes of protecting members of the public, which again may not be consistent with the welfare principle (s.19). Where any court has made a supervision order in respect of a child, the mere fact that the child has been received into care will not affect the operation of the order (s.8(1)).

Emigration. The 1980 Act preserves the power of a local authority to arrange for the emigration of a child in its care, though this may only be done with the consent of the Secretary of State. He will only allow action to be taken where he is satisfied that emigration could benefit the child, that suitable arrangements for his reception and welfare in the country to which he is going have been made, and that, where practicable, parents or guardians have been consulted. The child must also consent, if old enough to express an opinion on the matter. If not, official consent may still be given provided the child is emigrating with a parent, guardian or relative, or is to join any of them abroad. This power can seldom be used for the purpose for which it was intended when passed, but is useful today to assist children to return to their countries of origin (s.24).

Education, training and after-care. The Act empowers local authorities to guarantee deeds of apprenticeship and articles of clerkship entered into by children in their care (s.23) and to give financial assistance towards the expenses of accommodation, maintenance, education or training of persons over the age of 17, who were, before that age, in the care of the local authority (s.27). In addition, a duty is imposed on the local authority to advise and befriend any children who have formerly been in the care of local authorities, except where their welfare does not require it (s.28(1)). Where a young person who was formerly in care up to the age of 17 and is still under 21, approaches the local authority, it has the power to visit, advise and befriend and in exceptional circumstances, to give financial assistance to that child (s.29).

Reviews. While a child remains in the care of the local authority then, notwithstanding the general duty to promote the welfare of the child throughout his childhood (s.18), it is also required to review the case of each child in accordance with regulations to be made by the Secretary of State (s.20). When originally introduced in 1969, this provision imposed an obligation to arrange reviews at six-monthly intervals but laid down no guidelines as to how they should be conducted. The Children Act 1975 thus required local authorities to review cases in accordance with regulations to be made by the Secretary of State, which would also prescribe the frequency of reviews. Since the Secretary of State has not made any regulations, this part of the section in the 1980 Act is still inoperative, and the governing provision remains that in the Children and Young Persons Act 1969 (s.27(4)), so that reviews should take place every six months.

It is the duty of the local authority to safeguard and promote the interests of the child throughout his childhood, which clearly envisages long-term planning for the future of all children in care. Where prospects of rehabilitation within the natural family are bleak, children should not be kept waiting, condemned to spend the rest of their lives in a children's home, for pleasant though these may be they can never be a substitute for a permanent home with foster or adoptive parents (*Rowe and Lambert*, 1973). On the other hand, where prospects for rehabilitation are good, positive steps should be taken to ensure that the child does not spend longer in the children's home than is absolutely necessary. The six-monthly review is thus crucial. There has however been considerable criticism of the way in which such reviews are conducted (*N.C.B.*, 1977 and *B.A.A.F.*, 1980). The DHSS has suggested that, in cases where a child is fostered, the case conference should include the social worker with primary responsibility on the case, foster parents, parents and the child himself as well as more senior staff (*DHSS*, 1976). It is submitted that in cases where a child is in a residential home, the review should always include at least one member of the residential staff, who is, after all, standing in place of foster parents in the child's life.

The local authority obviously has the right to put its views forward at the review since it is charged with the responsibility of holding it (C.Y.P.A. 1969, s.27(4)) and the child also has the right to have his views considered (1980 Act, s.18). The child's parents, however, are not given the right to be present, nor if present the right to be heard or to have their views taken into account. Since the decisions made in these reviews may be of crucial importance to the child and his family, everyone who is to be affected should be able to participate fully in the discussion. The sorts of decision that can be made include the decisions to place a child with possible adoptive parents, the termination of parental contact, and even the placement of the child in secure accommodation. Although there are now procedures laid down whereby these last two types of decisions can be challenged in the courts, it is at least arguable that the minimal requirements of natural justice should be observed. Thus, everyone should be given the opportunity to express his views. This view does not commend itself to all commentators (*Hoggett*, 1981. On reviews more generally see *Sinclair*, 1983).

Medical treatment and death of child in care. The right to consent to medical treatment lies with the parent on behalf of the child, until he reaches 16. On admission into care and placement in a residential home, responsibility for the routine medical supervision will fall upon the local authority since the child is physically in their possession, and the Community Homes Regulations 1972 make provision for day to day medical care of children in the homes. Any major treatment however probably requires the consent of the parents where possible, and the 1972 Regulations provide for parents to be informed of any serious illness affecting the child, or of the outbreak of any serious illness in the children's home, which may then influence a parent's decision to remove the child from care.

Where a child in care dies, the authority is empowered to bury or cremate the body of the deceased child. The authority cannot, however, undertake cremation where such practice is not in accordance with the child's religion. Where the child is under 16, the parents may, if they are able to afford it, be asked to contribute to the funeral expenses. If the parent's income is insufficient to meet such expenses no contribution will be required, and if they need financial assistance to attend the child's funeral, the local authority has power to defray their expenses (s.25 and s.26).

Assumption of parental rights under the Child Care Act 1980, s.3

Where a child has been received into care under section 2 of the 1980 Act, on satisfaction of certain strictly defined conditions the local authority may assume parental rights in respect of that child. For some children this might occur early in their life in care, for others it should happen earlier than it often does, and for the rest their stay in care may be so short or for such reasons that such a step is unnecessary. It is important for all those concerned with the child to know if the authority has assumed parental rights since this materially affects the rights, duties and responsibilities exercisable by the authority and its staff.

A resolution may only be passed in respect of a child in care under section 2. It cannot be used to remove a child from his parents' home. Faced with a parent's demand for the immediate return of a child who has been in care for less than six months, it is unlikely that the local authority could achieve the passing of a resolution at such short notice, and thus alternative action such as wardship might possibly be considered.

The local social services committee cannot pass a resolution unless the conditions laid down in section 3 are met, and the decision to assume parental rights the most appropriate action in the circumstances. A proper investigation of the material facts should be conducted and the committee should not simply rubber-stamp the recommendations of the social workers (*Re D* (*a minor*), 1978), though it usually does. Before a resolution is passed the committee therefore must be satisfied that *one* of the conditions specified in section 3(1) is fulfilled:

(a) *that the child's parents are dead and he has no guardian or custodian (when Part II of the Children Act 1975 is eventually implemented);*

(b) *that the child's parent, guardian or custodian has:*

    (i) *abandoned him; or*

    (ii) *suffers from some permanent disability rendering him incapable of caring for the child; or*

    (iii) *while not falling within (ii)) suffers from a mental disorder, which renders him unfit to have the care of the child; or*

    (iv) *is of such habits or modes of life as to be unfit to have the care of the child; or*

    (v) *has so consistently failed without reasonable cause to discharge the obligations of a parent as to be unfit to have the care of the child; or*

(c) *that a resolution under ground (b) is in force in relation to one parent of the child, who is, or is likely to become a member of the household comprising the child and the other parent; or*

(d) *that throughout the three years preceding the passing of the resolution the child has been in the care of the local authority under section 2 or partly in the care of a local authority and partly in the care of a voluntary organisation (see further, Hoggett, 1981, Maidment, 1983).*

Wherever possible the assumption of parental rights by the local authority should not come like a bolt out of the blue to parents, child or residential staff. Good social work practice demands that the action has been fully discussed and that everyone appreciates the reasons for such action and sees it as a positive step for all concerned (*Adcock*, 1980). If the preparatory work is successful, parents may well consent to the resolution in writing, but where they have not done so, they must be informed of the passage of the resolution immediately by notice in writing. This notification will further inform the parents of their right to object by serving a written counter-notice within 14 days, which will automatically cause the resolution to lapse unless within that period the local authority refers the matter to the juvenile court for its consideration (s.3(3), (4), (5)). (See now B.A.A.F., 1983.)

The juvenile court will then have to decide whether the resolution should lapse, and to avoid this the local authority must satisfy the court of three conditions: that the original ground on which the resolution was passed was made out; that there are still grounds (though not necessarily the same one, *W.* v. *Nottinghamshire County Council*, 1981) on which the resolution could be passed; and that it is in the interests of the child that the resolution should not lapse (s.3(6)). In these proceedings the issue is clearly parental fitness; the argument is really between the local authority and the parents, although there is provision in the Act for the appointment of a guardian ad litem and for the preparation of an independent welfare officer's report (the relevant section (s.7) came into force on May 27, 1984). Either side if unsuccessful may appeal to the Family Division of the High Court (see further, *Smith*, 1979).

The necessity for informing residential staff of the passage of a resolution in respect of a child is threefold. First, they may be able to give vital information to the social worker in charge of the case to support the assumption of parental rights, for example, where consistent failure (s.3(6)(v)) is alleged, evidence may be available of failure to keep access appointments. Secondly, and linked with the first, residential staff are increasingly being called as witnesses in proceedings in some parts of the country where the resolution is being challenged by the parents, and if this is to happen it is only fair that they should be fully in the picture. Thirdly, and probably from the child's point of view most important, residential staff should be fully informed so that they can help the child to adjust to the new situation, appreciate what it may mean, and also cope with the highly emotional behaviour in which parents, who cannot adjust to being judged wanting in that role or who simply feel guilty, may seek to indulge.

Consequences of a parental rights resolution

General. Assuming the parents do not object, or a juvenile court directs that the resolution should not lapse, what will be the legal consequences for all concerned? The resolution vests nearly all parental rights and duties solely in the local authority, unless the resolution was passed only in respect of one parent (as in ground (b)) and she had parental rights with another parent, in which case the authority will exercise parental rights jointly with that parent (s.3(1)). A section 3 resolution continues in force until the child in respect of whom it was passed attains the age of 18, unless it is earlier rescinded by a resolution of the local authority (s.3(3)) or determined by order of the court upon a complaint being made (s.3(4)). A resolution also ceases to be effective if the child is adopted or where a guardian of the child is appointed by the court (s.3(2) and G.M.A. 1971, s.5).

Exactly what is meant by the phrase "parental rights" has never been satisfactorily defined by statute, but section 3 attempts a limited definition for its own purposes which is exclusive rather than inclusive in character (s.3(10)). Thus, the statute provides that the parental rights and duties which the authority will acquire do *not* include the right to consent or refuse to consent to an adoption freeing application or the right to agree or refuse to agree to the making of an adoption order (s.3(10)). The new provisions of the Child Care Act 1980, ss.12A–G (inserted by H. & S.S. & S.S.A.A. 1983, s.6 and Sched. I) further make it clear that although the local authority has the power to control arrangements for access to children in care by their parents, it does not have the right to terminate such access in relation to section 3 children without the parents being able to appeal to the courts (C.C.A. 1980, s.12A). No further assistance as to the scope of parental rights and duties acquired by the authority is given. Resort must therefore be made to the only other statutory provision which attempts a definition, and thence necessarily to the scope of the phrase at common law, both of which have attracted attention from several commentators (see *Hall*, 1972; *Thomson*, 1974; *Eekelaar*, 1973; *Maidment*, 1981; *Freeman*, 1982).

In the Children Act 1975, it is provided that the phrase "parental rights and duties" means as respects a particular child (whether legitimate or not) "all the rights and duties which by law the mother and father have in relation to a legitimate child and his property; and reference to a parental right or duty shall be construed accordingly and shall include a right of access and any other element included in a right or duty" (C.A. 1975, s.85(1)). The concept of parental rights and duties thus remains vague and imprecise, and though the writers referred to above have all attempted to draw up lists of such rights, they are by no means in agreement as to which passes to the local authority by virtue of a resolution, and which may remain in the parent. What does seem clear, even from a perusal of the statute, is that section 3(1) is not quite as all-embracing as it might at first appear. By no means are all parental rights and duties passed by virtue of the resolution to the local authority. Even without the complication of a resolution splitting these rights (see above) at least one judge has admitted that "if one were asked to define what are the rights of a parent àpropos his child, I for one would find it very difficult." (Ormrod J. in *Re N.*, 1974).

In relation to the rights and duties which the local authority acquire as the result of a resolution, and those which the parents retain, the principles set out below (a)–(d) can be stated with some certainty. The authority cannot cause a child to be brought up in any religious creed other than that in which he would have been brought up but for the resolution (s.4(3)). The Community Homes Regulations 1972 further provide that the child's religious beliefs should be respected.

(a) *Parental contact and access.* It is the parents who are placed under a duty to keep in touch with the local authority and to inform it of their whereabouts (C.C.A. 1980, s.9) though regrettably the authority is under no duty to tell parents the whereabouts of their child. It is now clear that local authorities have the right to make and control arrangements with regard to access to children in their care by parents, (see above, pp. 29–30) but the right to terminate such rights of access is subject to an appeal by the parents to the courts in the case of children who are the subject of a parental rights resolution (C.C.A. 1980, s.12A(1)(*h*)).

Where a local authority proposes to terminate the parents' right of access or to refuse to make arrangements for such access, it must first give the parent, guardian or custodian notice of such termination or refusal in a form prescribed by order made by the Secretary of State (s.12B(1)). The notice must inform the parent, guardian or custodian of the right to apply to a court for an order under section 12C, and where the notice purports to terminate access this takes effect as from the date of service. The notice must either be delivered personally, or left at or posted to the parents' proper address (s.12B(6)). Where a notice under section 12B has been served on the parent he may then apply by way of complaint to an appropriate juvenile court for an access order (s.12C(1) and (2)). An access order is an order requiring the authority to allow the child's parent, guardian or custodian access to the child subject to such conditions as the order may specify with regard to commencement, frequency, duration or place of access or to any other matter for which it appears to the court that provision ought to be made in connection with the requirement to allow access (s.12C(3)). Any decision which the juvenile court makes in relation to access orders is subject to a right of appeal in all parties to the High Court (s.12C(5)). Once an access order has been made a parent, guardian, custodian or the local authority may apply to the court for the variation or discharge of any such order (s.12D). Special powers are given to a single justice of the peace, who is a member of the juvenile court panel, to issue an emergency order suspending access for a period of up to seven days where he is satisfied that continued access to a child by its parent, guardian or custodian in accordance with an access order would put the child's welfare seriously at risk (s.12E). Any court considering an application for an access order, or an appeal, or application to vary or discharge such an order is directed to regard the welfare of the child as the first and paramount consideration in determining the matter (s.12F(1)). This direction must also mean that the local authority in issuing any termination notice will also have had to regard the welfare of the child as the first and paramount consideration, which contrasts with its duty under section 18 of the Child Care Act 1980 to regard it as only the first consideration (see above, p. 32). The court is further empowered, where it considers it necessary in order to safeguard the interests of the child, to order that the child be made a party to the proceedings and have his interests represented by a guardian ad litem, who will in performing his duties be subject to rules of court yet to be issued (s.12F(2), (3), and (4)).

It is also provided in the statute (s.12G) that the Secretary of State shall prepare and from time to time revise, a code of practice with regard to access to children in care, and before preparing such code consult such bodies as appear to him concerned. Many would argue that such a code is long overdue but it remains to be seen how long it actually takes the Secretary of State to issue such a code. In the meantime however these new provisions allowing parents whose rights of access have been terminated, to appeal to the courts, marks a major step forward.

(b) *Property and succession rights.* Somewhat surprisingly perhaps the right to administer the child's assets and income may pass to the local authority, including the rights of succession to property (s.3(10)); thus if the child dies intestate the local authority may be entitled to his estate. If only one parent's rights have been assumed the authority and other parent would take in equal shares. Several writers (*Bevan and Parry*, 1975 and *Freeman*, 1981) have remarked on how strange this is, especially where the resolution has been passed not on the grounds of the parents' culpability but their disability. Maidment (1981) comments that whilst such a step is right at the stage of adoption it is scarcely appropriate at this earlier stage, and one of us has argued that the position is morally unjust. (*Freeman*, 1980).

The appointment of a testamentary guardian however is a right which remains with the parent and is unaffected by the passage of the resolution. What the position of such a guardian would be were the parents to die is somewhat unclear. Since no resolution is in force with respect to him, arguably he would be in the position of exercising parental rights and duties with the local authority.

(c) *Disputed rights.* Two areas of doubt remain; those of the parental right to consent to marriage, and the right to change the child's name. Do either of these rights pass to the local authority by virtue of the resolution?

On the issue of the right to consent to marriage some writers (*Maidment*, 1981 and *Lowe and White*, 1979) have argued that the right must pass. Certainly, registrars require the consent of the local authority if a child is in care under the 1980 Act and parental rights have been assumed under section 3. However, the Marriage Act 1949 (s.3 and Sched. 2) makes no provision for such consent to be obtained even as amended by the Children Act 1975. Th. consents referred to in these Acts as being required, are those of parents or guardians (and when in force custodians) alone, and other writers (*Freeman*, 1980 and *Hoggett*, 1981) doubt whether this right does pass to the local authority.

A stronger argument may be made out for the local authority's right to change a child's name, although again there is no consensus of view. There is also no clear statutory provision to put the matter beyond doubt. Whilst it is true that the Enrolment of Deeds (Change of Name) Amendment Regulations 1979 allow a local authority to make a declaration on behalf of a child, so that his name can be changed this merely gives the authority a *power* to do something on behalf of the child, not a *right* to do so. Thus, if the parents object, an application in wardship might be sought to prevent the change of name being effected. See *Hoggett*, 1981 for the opinion that a court would be most reluctant to allow a local authority to change a child's name.

(d) *Possession, care and control*. All those provisions formerly described as applicable to children in care under section 2, including such matters as access, restriction of liberty, after-care and medical care, and reviews apply also to children after the passage of a parental rights resolution.

The local authority's powers to control the child's movements when a resolution has been passed however are greater than where the child is simply in care under section 2. Thus, when the authority allows the child to be under the charge or control of his parent or guardian for a fixed period (s.21(2)) and then serves notice on the parents requiring the child's return (s.14) the parents must return the child or they commit a criminal offence (s.14). In addition the statute empowers the authority to seek a summons ordering that the child be returned to it (s.15(2)) and if necessary the issuing of a warrant to search premises in which the authority believe a child is being kept (s.15(3)). Failure to comply with the summons could give rise to a conviction and a fine not exceeding £100 (s.15(4)).

Heavier penalties also exist for those who assist children, who are the subject of a parental rights resolution, to run away from the care of the local authority. Such penalties also apply to those, who without lawful authority remove a child, or knowingly harbour or conceal a child who has run away or who prevent him from returning to the care of the local authority. Thus, a parent or other person found guilty of such conduct will be liable to a fine not exceeding £400 or to imprisonment for a term not exceeding 3 months or both (s.16(4)). Where however, a child is in care under section 2, and a resolution has been passed under section 3 in respect of only one parent, the other does not commit a criminal offence in taking away the child.

A local authority has the same powers to punish a child as anyone else having the care of the child, namely: the right lawfully to chastise him (C.Y.P.A. 1933, s.1(7)). Where the child is in a residential home this power is further restricted by the applicable regulations (see p. 64).

2. Children in care of local authority following removal from unsuitable adoptive or foster-care surroundings

The power exists under both the Foster Children Act 1980 (s.12) and the Adoption Act 1958 (s.43(3)) for the local authority to apply to the court for an order that a child being kept in unsuitable surroundings be removed to a place of safety. The authority *may* then decide to receive the child into their care under section 2 of the 1980 Act, though they are *not* under a duty to do so, and they should where practicable inform the parents of the removal. The grounds for reception into care are thus different from the ordinary section 2 grounds but it would appear that the consent of the parents is still necessary. Where consent is given, the child will be in care as under section 2 and the local authority will have the section 2 powers and duties. The provisions do not however make it clear whether the parents can remove their children at will.

3. Children in care following closure of a voluntary home

Where the Secretary of State orders a local authority to remove a child from a voluntary home which is not registered, or the registration of which is being cancelled, the local authority is under a duty to receive into section 2 care any children living in the home, even though the section 2 grounds do not exist (Child Care Act 1980, s.57(6)). The statute does not make it clear whether parental agreement is necessary, nor whether parents are able to remove their children, nor whether the notice provisions must later be complied with should the child remain with the local authority for more than six months. In all other respects the child may be treated as if in care under section 2.

4. Children committed into care of local authorities

Children may also be committed into the care of the local authority in a variety of other proceedings which may be of direct or indirect concern to them, but the outcome of which may materially affect their lives. The proceedings in which such committal orders can be made, and their consequences will therefore be discussed separately and, where, relevant reference will be made to earlier discussion.

(a) *Under guardianship legislation*

Where an application is made to a court by a parent for custody or access to a child, under the procedure laid down in section 9 of the Guardianship of Minors Act 1971, and the court considers that there are exceptional circumstances making it impracticable or undesirable for the minor to be entrusted to either of the parents or anyone else, the court may commit the care of the child to a specified local authority (the Guardianship Act 1973, s.2(2)(*b*)). Proceedings are usually taken under section 9 when the parents are in dispute over some aspect of the child's custody or upbringing, or for example, where the father of an illegitimate child decides to apply for custody or access.

An order committing the child into the care of the local authority under these provisions ceases to have effect when the child reaches 18 (1971 Act, s.11A(3)) and cannot in any event be made where the child is already 17 (G.A. 1973, s.4(2A)). The order can be varied or discharged by a subsequent order of the court on the application of a parent, guardian or local authority (G.A. 1973, s.4(3A)).

The effect of the order is that whilst it remains in force the child continues in the care of the local authority notwithstanding any claim by a parent or guardian. (G.A. 1973, s.4(5)). The legislation provides that the authority has all the powers and duties described in relation to children in care under section 2, subject to the exceptions specifically excluded by the statute, (G.A. 1973, s.4(4)). Thus, where the committal order was made by the High Court only, then the exercise by the local authority of their powers to restrict the child's liberty, or to direct where he shall live (1980 Act, ss.18 and 21) shall be subject to any directions given by the court. In addition where the committal to care is made under guardianship legislation the local authority cannot arrange for the child's emigration, provide any after-care services, or take proceedings for contribution orders. Parents remain under a duty to maintain their children when in care but this is enforced by the making of a maintenance order in the guardianship proceedings (see p. 89). Except where the committal order is made by the High Court it seems that the local authority will have the power to control parental contact with the child. The parent is under a duty to keep in touch with the authority who are in turn empowered to assist with visiting expenses.

(b) *Under adoption or custodianship legislation*

Virtually identical provisions apply to a child who is committed to care following a court's refusal to make an adoption order (Children Act 1975, s.17). The ground for making the order is the same and the provisions of the guardianship legislation relating to the powers of the local authority are specifically incorporated in the Children Act (s.17). The local authority thus has all the powers described in relation to the guardianship provisions, with the same exceptions applying where the committal order was made by the High Court, when the local authority will again be subject to directions on major decisions from the High Court.

The position is exactly the same in respect of the revocation of a custodianship order (Children Act 1975, s.36) though as yet the power even to make these orders is not in force. Again the relevant provisions of the guardianship legislation are specifically incorporated and where the High Court revokes the order it will retain the power to issue directions.

(c) *Committal to care in matrimonial proceedings*

Whilst guardianship proceedings can be used by parents to settle any disputes which they have over their children, the primary concern in matrimonial proceedings is resolution of the many problems arising from the breakdown of the parents' relationship. Though there may be sympathy with the parents' predicament, the chief casualties are often the children, for the adults should be old enough to look after themselves.

In matrimonial proceedings, provision exists to allow the courts to commit children into the care of the local authority on dealing with the issue of their custody, on exactly the same grounds as are required under the guardianship legislation. The consequences of the making of such orders differ only marginally depending on the proceedings used. There is evidence to suggest that an increasing number of children are being committed to care in matrimonial proceedings chiefly under the divorce legislation, a result directly attributable to the rising divorce rate (*DHSS*, 1982).

Where the child is committed into the care of the local authority *by the magistrates' courts* under its powers in the Domestic Proceedings and Magistrates' Courts Act 1978 (ss.8(2) and 10) the effect is exactly the same as for an order under the guardianship legislation but the court, not being a High Court, does not retain any power to give directions as to major decisions affecting the child's life. Thus, as far as these children are concerned, the local authority has the power to regulate access and to terminate parental contact, subject to the rights of appeal described earlier (see above, p. 40) and subject to the exceptions applicable in guardianship cases the child can be treated as a section 2 child.

The authority is not given quite such wide-ranging powers in relation to children committed into their care *by the divorce courts* in divorce proceedings under the terms of section 43 of the Matrimonial Causes Act 1973. The basis for the order being made is the same as that for an order under the guardianship legislation and the restrictions on the local authority's powers almost identical. In the case of children committed in divorce proceedings however, whichever court makes the committal order retains the power to give directions on matters concerning the care and control of the children (M.C.A. 1973, s.43(5)). So any decisions as to access or termination of parental contact, or any other major decision affecting the child should in practice be referred back to the divorce court (and see *Re R.*, 1983).

(d) *Committal to care in wardship*

In certain circumstances parents, relatives, the local authority or any other interested person may apply to the High Court to have a child made a ward of court (Supreme Court Act 1981, s.41). Where an application is successful, the child is placed under the protection of the court and it must decide on the best future course of action for the child. The Family Law Reform Act 1969 provides in virtually identical form to the guardianship and matrimonial legislation that in exceptional circumstances an order can be made committing the child to the care of the local authority (s.7(2)).

The child remains a ward of court until it reaches the age of 18, unless the court on the application of anyone interested thinks that it should be discharged at an earlier stage. Any order committing the child to the care of the local authority remains in force until discharged by order of the court.

The effects of the committal order are that the child is to be treated as if it had been received into care under section 2, though while the order continues in force the child remains in care, notwithstanding any claim by the parent or guardian, or any other person. The other provisions relating to children committed to care by a divorce court apply equally to children committed to care in wardship (F.L.R.A. 1969, s.7(2) and (3)). The wardship court jealously guards its powers to give directions as to the upbringing of the child (s.7(3) incorporation, M.C.A. 1973, s.43(5)). It is clear from *Re Y* (1975) and *Re R* (1983) that this includes a power to give specific orders governing access, and from *Re C.B.* (1981), the power to veto any decision made by the local authority to move a child from one foster home to another.

5. Care orders and remand orders made under the Children and Young Persons Act 1969

(i) *General*

The circumstances in which children may be made the subject of a care order by the juvenile court are to be found in sections 1(1), 7 and 15 of the 1969 Act. Leaving aside the offence ground (s.1(1)(*f*)), the grounds contained in section 1 deal predominantly with situations where the child is the victim, section 7 deals with the child as a threat, and section 15 covers both possibilities. Proceedings under section 1 are civil, those under section 7 criminal and under section 15 may be either. Where a child is remanded to the care of the local authority, this occurs in the course of criminal proceedings (s.23(1)). While the circumstances in which the care or remand order is made may differ, the consequences are indistinguishable and are in many instances identical to those where the child is in care under section 2 of the Child Care Act 980.

The only exception to this general principle is that where the local authority makes any attempt to terminate a parent's right of access to a child in the care of the local authority under these provisions, the procedure laid down under sections 12B–H of the Child Care Act 1980 must be followed (s.12A(1)(*a*) and (*c*) and for that procedure see above, p. 40).

(ii) *Care orders under Children and Young Persons Act 1969, s.1*

Care proceedings are generally commenced at the instance of the local authority though the Police and the N.S.P.C.C. may also initiate proceedings, and where the education ground is relied upon then the education authority is solely responsible. Wherever the initiator is not the local authority, it must be informed and, where the child is over 12, the probation department should also be told. If a local authority is advised that a child might be at risk it is under a duty to investigate the circumstances unless it considers it unnecessary, and must commence proceedings where there appear to be grounds for the making of a care order. Before proceedings for a full care order are commenced the same circumstances may have already formed the basis for the making of an interim care order (s.2(10)), the making of a place of safety order (s.28(1)) or a police place of safety order (s.28(2)) but this does not prevent the same evidence being used again.

The section 1 grounds are in two limbs, primary grounds and a secondary proviso, both of which must be established to the satisfaction of the court before a care order may be made. The primary grounds include a list of seven conditions, any one of which must be proved, and a secondary proviso, the care or control condition, which must also be satisfied. The seven primary conditions need only be established on the balance of probabilities. They are:

*(a) the child's proper development is being avoidably pre-
vented or neglected or his health is being avoidably impaired or
neglected or he is being ill-treated*

This ground not only covers children who are the victims of deli-
berate child abuse but it extends to other situations in which
parents may not be so obviously responsible for their child's failure
to develop (*Hoggett*, 1981). Exactly what is meant by proper
development is problematic, but at least one High Court judge has
indicated that it not only emcompasses physical but also mental
and emotional development (*F*. v. *Suffolk County Council*, 1981).
The present tense is used throughout the subsection so an authority is unable to rely on it where it fears for the future safety of a
child (*Essex County Council* v. *TLR and KBR*, 1978). It may do so
however if the ground can be proved to have existed when the
parent last had the care and control of the child in the chain of
events immediately preceding the issue of a summons (*H*. v. *Shef-
field City Council*, 1981).

*(b) it is probable that the first ground will be satisfied in this
child's case having regard to the fact that the court or another
court has found that the ground is or was satisfied in the case of
another child or young person who is or was a member of the
household to which the child belongs*

So, where other children have been the victims of abuse or neglect, whether or not they were ever the subjects of care proceedings, a sibling also thought to be at risk may be protected (*Surrey
County Council* v. *S.*, 1974). The probability of harm must have
existed for the child in question before a care order will be made
on this ground.

*(bb) it is probable that the conditions in (a) will be satisfied in
this child's case having regard to the fact that a person who has
been convicted of an offence mentioned in Schedule 1 to the
1933 Act including a person convicted of such an offence on
whose conviction for the offence an order was made under Part
1 of the Powers of Criminal Courts Act 1973 placing him on
probation or discharging him absolutely or conditionally is, or
may become, a member of the same household as the child or
young person.*

This ground covers conviction for an offence against any child or young person, and the list of offences contained in the schedule is quite extensive. Generally known as the "Kepple clause," this is a complete misnomer for William Kepple, Maria Colwell's stepfather, had no convictions for violence against children or young persons; thus, the clause would have been useless as protection for a child in similar circumstances to those of Maria. The addition by virtue of the H.&S.S.&S.S.A.A. 1983 of a person who upon conviction has received only a probation order or a discharge plugs a gap in the protection which many thought vital. (*B.A.A.F.*, 1980).

(c) he is exposed to moral danger

This ground is not widely used. It can cover exposure to sexual immorality, to the risks of drug addiction and anything else which could reasonably be deemed to be morally dangerous. Where sexual abuse within the family is suspected, this ground is clearly the most suitable though institutional care does not necessarily guarantee protection from such abuse (see *Kincora*, 1982). There may also be some difficulty in determining the conventional morality by which the behaviour to which the child is exposed is to be judged (*Mohamed* v. *Knott*, 1969).

(d) he is beyond the control of his parent or guardian

It is under this ground that the parents can approach the local authority and ask them to take some action, more usually when they have exhausted all their own powers of criticism, punishment and restraint. Hoggett (1981) also suggests that it can be useful where the child is guilty of offences such as petty theft, but because of the child's age (*i.e.* under ten) he cannot be dealt with under any other measure.

(e) he is of compulsory school age and is not receiving efficient full-time education suitable to his age, ability and aptitude

Responsibility for bringing proceedings on this ground lies with the local education authority (s.2(8)) but non-attendance may also have been symptomatic of other problems, which may have led to a care order being sought on other grounds, for example ground (a).

(f) he is guilty of an offence excluding homicide

This ground had been rarely used prior to 1983 because the procedure available under section 7(7) had not, until the implementation of the Criminal Justice Act 1982, required anything other than a conviction in criminal proceedings (see below, pp. 51–52). Where a child is dealt with in care proceedings, however, his position will now be no different from that in which he would have been if prosecuted (C.Y.P.A. 1969, s.3). In addition, the court cannot be satisfied that the ground is established unless the child would have been found guilty in criminal proceedings.

Once the primary ground has been established, the court must then be satisfied on the secondary ground, *that the child is in need of care or control which he is unlikely to receive unless the court makes an order.*

When satisfied on both these limbs, the court may, *if it thinks fit,* make a care order. The court should therefore have been convinced that such an order is the best possible solution for the child in its particular circumstances. Although in care proceedings the initial stages will be concerned with proving the grounds rather than with the welfare of the child, when it is deciding how to dispose of the child, the court in exercising its discretion should have regard to the welfare of the child (C.Y.P.A. 1933, s.44(1)) emphasised in *Re S.*, 1978). Thus, if there is any chance that an order might do the child more harm than good—it should not be made, though the evidential burden on the person making such a suggestion may well be very difficult to discharge (*Re S*).

(iii) *Care orders under Children and Young Persons Act 1969, ss.7(7) and 15*

Where a juvenile is found guilty of a criminal offence which in the case of an adult could result in imprisonment, then by section 7(7)(A) (as inserted by C.J.A. 1982, s.23) the court can make a care order provided it is satisfied that such an order is appropriate because of the seriousness of the offence, and that the child or young person is in need of care or control which he is unlikely to receive unless the court makes a care order. The court cannot make such an order under section 7(7) in respect of a child or young person, who is not legally represented unless he has applied for and been refused legal aid, or having been informed of his right to do so, has failed or refused to apply (C.Y.P.A. 1969, s.7A). The effects of such a care order are exactly the same as those resulting from an order under section 1: thus the new procedures relating to termination of parental access apply in relation to these children (C.C.A. 1980, s.12A(1)(*a*) and see above, p. 40). Similarly, where a juvenile under 18 has previously been the subject of a supervision order, under section 15 a juvenile court on the application of the supervisor may discharge that order and substitute instead a care order, having the same consequences as those made under sections 1 and 7(7)(*a*). A court should only substitute a care order in those circumstances where it is satisfied that the supervised person is unlikely to receive the care and control which he needs (s.15).

(iv) *Charge and control orders*

In addition to the power to make ordinary care orders in respect of juvenile offenders, the courts now have a further power conferred by the Criminal Justice Act 1982 to make a charge and control order, which operates on top of the ordinary care order (C.Y.P.A. 1969, s.20A). This power can be used where a juvenile, who is already the subject of a care order because of an offence, is found guilty of another offence. Where this is proved, the court may impose a charge and control order to the effect that the child must not be allowed to return to the charge and control of any parent, guardian, relative or friend for a period of up to six months (s.20A(1)(*a*)) or to the charge and control of a specified parent, guardian, relative or friend for such similar period (s.20A(1)(*b*)). This order has somewhat misleadingly been referred to quite widely as a "residential care order" but this is to misunderstand the courts actual powers under the section. The court cannot direct that a child be held in local authority residential care: thus if the local authority chooses to board the child out with foster parents pursuant to the making of such an order, such action is not restricted by the order. The court should not exercise its powers to make an order unless it is of the opinion that no other method of dealing with the child is appropriate, and for deciding whether this is the case, the court should obtain and consider information about the child's circumstances (s.20A(3)). A charge and control order should also not be imposed without the child being given the opportunity to be legally represented, and if his means are such that he requires assistance, he will be eligible for legal aid (s.20A(4)). Where the order is imposed its effects and purposes must be fully explained to the child. At any time whilst the charge and control order is in force the child, parent acting on his behalf, or the authority may apply for variation or revocation (s.20A(6)), but if the child offends yet again during the currency of the order, a further charge and control order may be imposed (s.20A(2)).

The local authority and the child have the power to appeal to the Crown Court against the imposition of a charge and control order or its terms. (s.20A(7)).

Duration of care orders. Care orders last until the juvenile attains the age of 18 unless aged 16 at the time of the order in which case it lasts until he is 19 (s.20(3)). The Act also provides that the local authority can apply for an order which would otherwise lapse at 18 to extend to 19, where the child is in a community home or youth treatment centre, and should be kept there for his own or the public's sake because of his mental condition or behaviour (s.21(1)). The child (s.21(2)), his parents (s.70(2)) or the authority may at any time apply for the discharge of the order, but where such an application is unsuccessful it cannot be repeated in under three months unless the court gives its consent (s.21(3)(*b*)). (See further, *Smith*, 1979 and *Feldman*, 1978).

Effects of care orders. Despite the very different reasons for the imposition of a care order in respect of a child, there are few differences in the legal effects of such orders. The principal effect of a care order is that it imposes a duty on the local authority to receive the child into its care and notwithstanding any claim by his parent or guardian, to keep him in their care while the order is in force (Child Care Act 1980, s.10(1)). The local authority has virtually the same powers and duties with respect to a child in their care as they have in respect of children in care under section 2 of the 1980 Act, with certain clearly defined exceptions (see, *e.g.* C.C.A. 1980, s.12A, above, p. 28). In addition because of the local authority's duty to keep the child despite parental demands for his return, provisions relating to the arrest of a child who absconds, and prosecution for various offences of assisting the child similar to those which will apply in relation to children who are the subject of parental rights resolutions, are to be found in the 1980 Act (s.16). Identical provisions apply where the child is the subject of a remand order under section 23(1) or is being detained in the care of the authority under section 29(3) (see below).

Exercise of parental powers, rights and duties. Where the child is in care under a care order the authority has the same powers in relation to the accommodation and maintenance of the child, the medical and dental care of the child, the emigration of the child, the imposition of discipline and restriction of the child's liberty as it had in relation to a child in care under section 2 of the 1980 Act. The local authority is able to control access to a child in care under these provisions but where it takes steps to terminate such access or refuses to make arrangements, it will be subject to the appeals procedure laid down in section 12A of the Child Care Act 1980 (see above p. 40).

The authority has duties similar to those which are exercisable in relation to children in care under section 2, but who are also the subject of parental rights resolutions. The primary duty imposed by section 18 thus applies to all children in the care of the local authority, and as with the other children the local authority is under a duty to review the care of each child in their care at six-monthly intervals (see above, pp. 33–34). In addition in the case of a care order child the authority must consider, in the course of the review, whether an application should be made for the discharge of the order (C.Y.P.A. 1969, s.27(4)). Where a child over the age of five, who is subject to a care order, has not been allowed to leave the community home to attend school or work for a period in excess of three months, and there has been little or no parental contact, the authority is under a further duty to appoint an independent visitor. The visitor's duties are to advise, visit and befriend the child, and if they think it necessary to apply on the child's behalf for discharge of the care order. The idea behind this provision is to afford the children some protection against the wide powers of the local authority, where they apparently have no one else to represent their interests. The conditions for eligibility for appointment as visitors are laid down by the Children and Young Persons (Definition of Independent Persons) Regulations 1971 and the 1969 Act, the Regulations and Official guidance make it quite clear that no one in any way connected with a community home should be appointed as a visitor nor any currently serving magistrates since this could lead to a conflict of duties (*Home Office*, 1971).

As with children in care under section 2 who are the subjects of parental rights resolutions, the authority must not cause a child in their care by virtue of a care order, to be brought up in any religious creed other than that in which he would have been brought up but for the order (s.10(3)). Similarly, where the child is in a residential home the regulations provide for the child's religious beliefs to be respected and wherever possible promoted.

Where their child is in care under a care order parents remain under a duty to contribute to their child's maintenance (s.45(1)) and to keep the local authority informed of their whereabouts and of any change of address (s.12). Should the local authority at any time decide that the child be removed from a residential home and placed somewhere with a view to adoption, the parents still retain the right to agree to or refuse to agree to the subsequent making of an adoption order (Adoption Act 1958, s.4(3)(*a*)).

(v) *Children who are subject to interim care orders and remand orders*

The provisions just described as applicable to care order children apply with equal force to those children who are in the care of the local authority under an interim care order or who have been remanded into its care, pending trial or sentence by the juvenile or Crown court (C.Y.P.A. 1969, ss.2(10) and 23(1)). Whilst the authority is therefore authorised to keep the child notwithstanding any claim by its parent or guardian, (C.C.A. 1980, s.10(1)) it is nonetheless under a duty to deliver the child up to enable the criminal process to be completed (s.10(4)).

Where a child who has been remanded to the care of the local authority under section 23 proves to be of such unruly character that he cannot continue to be housed in the local authority home to which he had been sent, the authority can apply to a court for a certificate of unruly character, and the child will be committed if possible to a remand centre, or failing this to prison (s.23(3)).

Regulations issued pursuant to section 69 of the Children Act 1975 prohibit the certification of girls under the age of 17 as unruly and boys over 15 can only be designated as unruly if:

(a) charged with an offence carrying a maximum sentence in the case of an adult of more than 14 years; or

(b) charged with an offence of violence or has previous convictions for violence;

(c) he has been previously living in a community home from which he has persistently absconded, or which he has seriously disrupted.

The conditions therefore which must be satisfied before a young person may be remanded under a certificate of unruliness are defined, but unruliness itself is not defined. It is thus up to the court to be satisfied both that one or more of the conditions above is fulfilled and that the degree of unruliness is such as to meet the requirements of section 23 of the 1969 Act (*Home Office*, 1977).

II. *Children in Care of Voluntary Organisations*

In practice these days, most of the children in children's homes run by voluntary organisations, other than those for mentally handicapped children, will be in the care of the local authority under the provisions already discussed. The local authority will then have placed the child in the care of the voluntary organisation, which has actual custody of the child but the local authority retains overall control. Where the child has not been placed by the local authority, voluntary organisations may possess similar powers to those held by an authority in relation to children in their care, though some of these are only exercisable with the assistance of others.

Where a child has been in the care of a voluntary organisation for more than six months, parents are under a duty to give 28 days notice to the organisation of their intention to remove the child, and failure to do so renders them guilty of a criminal offence (C.C.A. 1980, s.63). The Act thus applies the provisions of section 13 (see above, p. 32) to children in the care of voluntary organisations. The organisation therefore has 28 days breathing space in which either to approach the local authority in order to ask that parental rights and duties be transferred to the organisation, or to take steps to have the child made a ward of court. Where the organisation suspects that the authority might not take any action, or that the relevant grounds for a resolution could not be established, and it is seriously worried about the child, wardship will be the only step to be taken.

When it is necessary therefore, and not only in an emergency provoked by a parental demand for the child's return, the local authority has the power under section 64(1) to pass a resolution vesting in the organisation the parental rights and duties with respect to any child in the organisation's care. This action can only be taken where the child is not in the care of the local authority, the grounds for such a resolution exist (see above, pp. 36–37), and where it can be proved that such a step is necessary in the interests of the welfare of the child. Similarly, at any later stage if the authority thinks it necessary in the interests of the child, it can resolve that the parental rights and duties shall cease to be vested in the organisation and shall instead be vested in them (s.65).

Unless a subsequent resolution is passed transferring the rights and duties back to the local authority, the resolution lasts for exactly the same length of time as one passed under section 3 (see above, p. 38). The Act does however give parents the same rights of objection to the local authority against such resolutions, and rights of complaints to the juvenile court and of appeal to the High Court as they have under ordinary section 3 resolutions (s.67 and see above, p. 37). In all major respects the Act provides that such resolutions are identical in their effects to those passed by the local authority in favour of themselves. All the parental rights and duties, which a local authority has or is thought to have when in a similar position (see above, pp. 38–43), vest in the organisation in whose care the child is when the resolution is passed, subject to the statutory exceptions. The parents remain under a duty to keep the organisation informed of their whereabouts (s.64). The local authority by vesting parental rights and duties in the voluntary organisation does not entirely divest itself of all its responsibilities to the child. Thus, it can withdraw the resolution and transfer rights and duties to itself where the welfare of the child demands it (s.65); it must cause children in voluntary homes to be visited to ensure their well-being (s.68) and they are also under a duty to ensure the after-care of children in their area who have formerly been in the care of a voluntary organisation (s.69). These last two duties apply whether or not a resolution under section 65 has ever been passed. Many voluntary organisations further have the power and the resources under the terms of their foundation deeds to provide after-care for children formerly in their care, and where necessary financial assistance to help the child in any further training or education he proposes to undertake. In addition to the duties specifically imposed by the 1980 Act, the staff of the voluntary organisation running the residential home where the child is accommodated, are subject to the requirements laid down in the Administration of Children's Homes Regulations 1951, or the Community Homes Regulations 1972, whichever is applicable.

III. *Children in Care of Special Schools or Long-stay Hospitals*

(a) In special schools

Where a child is being educated at a special residential school he may also be in the care of the local authority under one of the many provisions previously described. Thus, if a parent approaches the local authority for assistance because he can no longer cope with a handicapped child, this can count as "any other circumstance" preventing the parent looking after the child, and so constitute grounds for a section 2 reception into care (see above, p. 26). The allocation of functions as between the care authority and the education authority is provided for in section 30 of the 1980 Act, including provision for the determination of liability for maintenance in respect of the child.

In some cases however, the child will not technically be "in care" and the special residential school, the local education authority and the parents will all have some powers and duties in respect of the child. This may occur for example where the parent approaches the local education authority under section 9 of the Education Act 1981 with a request for an assessment, the child is certified as requiring education in a special residential school and there is no need at all for any intervention by the local social services department.

Where a statement certifying the child's need has been issued under the Education Act 1981 and he has been registered at a special school, he cannot (even though not in the care of the local authority), be removed from that school by his parents without the consent of the local education authority (Education Act 1981, s.11(*a*)). The Act does not differentiate between day and boarding schools, so parents' rights are certainly curtailed to this extent. Where the child is a boarding pupil the staff at the school clearly have all the rights which go with having actual custody of the child, such as the right to punish the child (see above, p. 32). In other respects though since the child is not technically "in care," the parents retain all other rights and duties in respect of the child, except that if the placement in the boarding school was made by the local education authority, it is that authority who must pay the costs (see below p. 93).

Where a parent does wish to remove a child not in care from a special school, under section 11(2) of the Education Act 1981, the matter may be referred to the Secretary of State for Education, who can give such direction as he thinks fit. There is no provision for an appeal from the determination of the Secretary of State, but a parent who is seriously worried by the treatment which his child is receiving at a special school should issue wardship proceedings.

(b) In long-stay hospitals

Children who are not technically in care and who have become long-stay patients in a hospital are truly the forgotten children in terms of legislative protection. Because they are not "in care" no powers pass to the local authority, there is no duty to review their position, and while parents clearly retain all their rights and duties in respect of them, some never exercise them. Short of the child being abandoned, or the parents being deemed to have abandoned him, in which case the child could be received into care under section 2 (see above, p. 26) there is little that local authorities or even hospital staff can do to take over or to enforce the parents' duties in respect of his child. Where some positive action is required for the child's welfare, wardship may well be the only way to break the deadlock. Once the wardship court is appraised of the circumstances, it can make an order under the terms of section 7 of the Family Law Reform Act 1969 committing the care of the child to any individual or to the local authority. The person into whose care the child is committed will be subject to any directions of the court regarding the child's upbringing (s.7(3)).

IV. *Children in Care of Detention Centres, Borstals, Youth Custody Centres, Remand Centres or Prisons*

(a) Detention centre orders

A detention centre order can be made in respect of a child who has been convicted of a criminal offence, where imprisonment could be ordered for an adult for the same offence, and the offender is at least 14 years old (Criminal Justice Act 1982, s.4(1)). The period of detention can be anything from three weeks to four months (Criminal Justice Act 1982, s.4(2) and (4)). A detention order cannot be made in respect of girls, as there are no centres for them and none is planned (*DHSS*, 1980). Children in such centres are subject to the Detention Centre Rules 1983. The new detention centre order, like imprisonment, takes account of time spent in custody on remand (C.J.A. 1967, s.67(5)(*a*) as amended).

(b) Youth custody

Following implementation of the Criminal Justice Act 1982, the courts have been able instead of imposing sentences of borstal training to impose sentences of youth custody. The new sentence is served in designated training establishments and for offenders aged 17 or over but under 21 may be of four to 18 months in length and for offenders aged 15 and over may be of four to 12 months in length. Unlike sentences of borstal training, the new youth custody sentence like imprisonment takes account of time spent in custody on remand, and attracts one-third remission for offenders aged 17 and over. Any sentence in excess of four months applies equally to boys and girls aged 15 to 17, but whereas boys in that age group can in certain circumstances be given a shorter sentence (C.J.A. 1982, s.6(2) and s.7(6)) there is no similar power for the courts to exercise in relation to girls of the same age (C.J.A. 1982, s.6(4) and s.7(6) and see above, p. 24).

One final point to note in relation to youth custody sentences is that they cannot be suspended. Since the Criminal Justice Act 1982 provides that no court can pass a sentence of imprisonment on any person aged under 21 years this removes from the courts field of choice a valuable sentencing alternative in relation to young adult offenders. There were prior to the 1982 Act about 4,000 suspended sentences of imprisonment a year for young adults. As McEwan points out (1983) losing this measure (whatever the merits of introducing it in the first place) creates a grave risk of further adding to the numbers in youth custody centres and prison. (See further *Bottoms*, 1981). It is also not open to the court to partly suspend a sentence of youth custody.

(c) Children in remand centres and prisons

Children may find themselves in remand centres pending the outcome of criminal proceedings against them or where the local authority into whose care they had been committed have sought a certificate of unruly character from the court and have had them transferred to a remand centre (1969 Act, s.23(2)). A child may find himself in prison under exactly the same provisions. Following a direction in 1981 the minimum age at which boys can now be sent to remand centres or prisons under these provisions is 15. The responsibility for accommodating 14 year old boys on remand now falls on local authorities (*Home Office*, 1981).

(d) Children subject to detention

No sentence of imprisonment can be imposed in respect of a juvenile, but the Crown Court can in certain circumstances order a child to be *detained*. The place where the child is detained does not have to be a prison and can be such place as the Home Secretary directs (C.Y.P.A. 1933, s.53). The circumstances in which a sentence of detention can be imposed are where a child under 18 is convicted of murder, in which case they will be sentenced to be *detained* at *Her Majesty's Pleasure* (C.Y.P.A. 1933, s.53(1)); thus the sentence is indeterminate; and where a juvenile is convicted of an offence which in the case of an adult would attract a sentence of fourteen years or more, then the sentence must be no longer than that which would have been passed on an adult (C.Y.P.A. 1933, s.53(2)). Under the provisions of the Criminal Justice Act 1982 where a person aged 17 years or more but under the age of 21 is convicted of an offence other than murder, for which a person aged 21 years or over would be liable to imprisonment for life, the court shall, if it consider that a custodial sentence for life would be appropriate, sentence him to custody for life. (Criminal Justice Act 1982, s.8(2)).

(e) Effects of legal custody orders

A fortiori sentences of legal custody, whether detention centre orders, youth custody sentences or sentences of detention, operate in such a way that children are compulsorily removed from their parents' custody and placed in the actual custody of the particular penal establishment to which they have been sent. The parental rights and duties therefore which relate to the actual person of the child and including the right to determine access, pass to the establishment concerned subject to whatever sets of regulations apply to them (see below, pp. 78–81). No other parental rights or duties pass although the parents' liability to maintain the child is suspended for the period of the child's stay in a penal establishment. There is no power to order the parents to make contributions to the child's maintenance, and parents may lose their right to child benefit and other social security benefit increases.

V. *General Responsibility for acts of Children in Residential Care or Legal Custody*

Where a child in the care of the local authority or in legal custody commits a criminal offence then the authority or establishment in whose care the child is, is not deemed to be a parent or guardian for the purposes of section 55 of the Children and Young Persons Act 1933. (see *Leeds City Council* v. *West Yorkshire Police*, 1982). The law was confirmed by the Criminal Justice Act 1982 amending section 55 of the 1933 Act. Where the child does commit such a further offence while in care or in a penal establishment, the courts have all the usual powers to deal with him on a finding of guilt as if he were not in care or in custody (see above, pp. 51–52).

Similarly, the local authority or penal establishment (usually the Home Office) is not responsible for any tort which the juvenile commits, unless the opportunity arose as the result of negligence on the part of the establishment's staff. Even then, where the authority or establishment is acting in exercise of its statutory powers, it has been argued that liability to third parties should only arise where the exercise of the powers was manifestly unreasonable or made in bad faith. (*Home Office* v. *Dorset Yacht Co. Ltd.*, 1970). However, where a child of suspected arsonous tendencies escaped from a local authority community home where he was being held on remand charged with burglary and set fire to a local parish church, the local authority was held liable in damages in a negligence action. It was held to be so liable because one of its staff had known that the police suspected the child of two offences of arson but had failed to report these matters to the court or to the authority (*Vicar of Writtle* v. *Essex County Council*, 1979 and see *McEwan*, 1980).

3. Regulation of Residential Accommodation

I. *Regulation of Community Homes*

All community homes (see above, p. 13) whether they be local authority, controlled or assisted, are subject to the controls laid down in the Community Homes Regulations 1972. The power to make such regulations and to issue general guidance is, by virtue of the Child Care Act 1980 in the hands of the Secretary of State (s.39). The DHSS states in relation to these regulations that the general approach is to provide an up-to-date framework within which the responsible bodies will have the widest possible discretion in administering community homes (*DHSS*, 1972). The 1972 Regulations are therefore somewhat less detailed than the Administration of Children's Homes Regulations 1951 (see below, p. 70) and considerably less so than the former Approved School and Remand Home Rules which they replaced (*DHSS Advisory Council on Child Care*, 1971). Just occasionally though the 1972 Regulations go into greater detail than the former regulations on issues where experience has shown the need, or a fresh approach was thought desirable. Examples of this include the requirements for written reports on visits (reg. 3(2)); and for detailed records of disciplinary measures (reg. 10(4)).

General

The general principle to be observed by the body responsible for running the home is to be found in regulation 3. The responsible body must arrange for the community home to be conducted so as

63

to make proper provision for the care, treatment and control of the children who are accommodated therein. In furtherance of this aim regulations require monthly inspection visits of such homes and the submission of written reports consequent upon such visits.

Day-to-day care of children

The responsible body is charged with the task of ensuring that arrangements are made for providing adequate medical, dental and, where appropriate, psychiatric care for all children in the home, for maintaining satisfactory conditions of hygiene in the home, and for ensuring that adequate precautions are taken against fire and accidents, including the holding of drills. There is also a duty to provide suitable facilities for visits to the home by parents, guardians, relatives or friends of any of the children in residence. The times of visiting are within the discretion of the managers of the home, or with the local authority or its staff where it is a local authority home. The managers or persons in charge are also under a duty to notify the responsible body, the child's parents or guardians and the local authority in those circumstances where a child dies or suffers serious injury or illness.

Freedom of religion

The regulations provide that the managers or local authority must ensure that every child resident in the home has, so far as is practicable in the circumstances, the opportunity to attend such religious services and to receive such instruction as is appropriate to the religious pursuasion to which he may belong. The requirement is to provide the *opportunity*. The issue of whether corporate religious observance should be part of the normal routine in a given home is for the responsible body or managers to decide, but official guidance directs that if a child is of school age his regular attendance at school will normally constitute a sufficient discharge of the duty to provide the opportunity to receive religious instruction.

Control of children

The emphasis in the 1972 Regulations is much more on the maintenance of control within the home than on the punishment of children in marked contrast to the approach taken in the 1951 Regulations (see below, p. 70) and in the former Approved

School and Remand Home Rules which they replaced (*DHSS,* 1979). Thus, it is provided that control in the homes should be maintained on the basis of good personal and professional relationships between staff and children (*DHSS,* 1972). Further guidance is given on precisely what this means. It is stated that in the nature of things, good personal relationships in the home will come from respect for the individuality of children in it; while good professional relationships will involve the application of those special skills which enable the staff to cope with the problems associated with the child's removal from home. Such skills may include recognising and dealing sympathetically with behaviour directly attributable to the child's separation from his family, or by supplying a degree of support and encouragement and where necessary control, which is in the best interests of the child and the community. Research would seem to indicate that this is a very difficult balance for staff to maintain (*Wills,* 1971, *Cawson,* 1978). The regulations do however allow for stronger additional measures to be taken where they are considered necessary for the maintenance of control in the home, though such measures must be approved by the local authority. In approving any measure the authority is under a duty to have regard to the purpose and character of the home and the categories of children for which it is provided (see *Wills,* 1971). The approval must be given in writing and reviewed yearly, the regulations further providing that a complete and detailed record must be kept in the home of all occasions on which recourse is made to the additional measures. The DHSS stresses that the regulations do not specifically mention corporal punishment, this being left to the discretion of the parties directly concerned, and express the hope that authorisations for the use of corporal punishment will be given sparingly and as a last resort, and that local authorities will consider at annual reviews, in the light of experience, whether it is still needed (*DHSS,* 1972).

Many authorities still allow corporal punishment in community homes despite official disapproval. (*S.T.O.P.P.,* 1981). It is arguable that the use of a cane in a community home is contrary to the welfare principle set out in section 18 of the Child Care Act 1980 (see above, pp. 33–34). The Secretary of State for Social Services in the last Labour Government let all Directors of Social Services know that he believed it to be undesirable and improper in a professional caring relationship. The Handicapped and Deprived

Children (Abolition of Corporal Punishment) Bill 1979 would have abolished the power to beat mentally handicapped, physically handicapped and deprived children but the Bill failed. There is considerably irony in the situation where a child can be removed from his parents' home because he is thought to be at risk of non-accidental injury only to be placed in a position where physical assaults on him are institutionally sanctioned. It could very well be argued that a community home caning is a non-accidental injury which ought to be entered on the "at-risk" register. Many children are on registers for much less. It is also ironical that Parliament has outlawed the taking of a photograph of a child being whipped when at the same time it refuses to outlaw the Act itself (Protection of Children Act 1978). There can be no justification for the retention of physical punishment in community homes and children in community homes should be immune from such abuse.

II. *Regulation of Secure Accommodation*

Only a small minority of community homes were originally envisaged as needing secure provision (*DHSS*, 1975). In the remainder staff were expected to and do rely on other sanctions to exercise control whether by the withholding of certain privileges or in more difficult cases, the administration of corporal punishment.

The number of secure places within the community homes system has certainly been on the increase in recent years, although the use of such units for difficult children varied enormously as between different local authorities. In 1980, 2000 children were at any one time in secure containment of one sort or another, (*House of Commons*, 1982). The DHSS had stated that attempts should be made to ensure the development within the community home system of units with places for several children so as to avoid isolation of the child and the strain on the staffing resources in ordinary homes. These factors had all led to calls for greater controls on the provision and use of secure accommodation, (*DHSS*, 1981; *Parliamentary Penal Affairs Group*, 1981; *Children's Legal Centre*, 1982), and beliefs that the provisions of section 24 of the Children and Young Persons Act 1969 might be held by the European Court of Human Rights as contravening the Convention in that children deprived of their liberty had no access to courts, forced the

Government into enacting the new section 21A of the Child Care Act 1980.

It is now provided (by C.J.A. 1982, s.25), that the liberty of a child in care should be restricted only if he has a *history* of absconding, *and* is likely to abscond if he is kept in some other kind of accommodation, *and* is likely to be at risk as to his physical, mental or moral welfare if he absconds; or if otherwise he is likely to injure himself or other persons (the new C.C.A. 1980, s.21A(1)). This section further enables the Secretary of State to make regulations providing for the conditions under which a child may be contained in secure accommodation and the duration of that containment in various circumstances. (C.C.A. 1980, s.21A(2)) Regulations issued pursuant to this power are the Secure Accommodation (No.2) Regulations (S.I. 1983 No. 1808) which came into force on January 1, 1984. The Regulations provide that any accommodation to be used for the purpose of restricting the liberty of children in community homes must be approved by the Secretary of State, (r.3). In line with the recommendations of the DHSS cited earlier, the accompanying circular indicates that the use of single secure rooms in community homes should be ended as soon as possible, and that no approval will be given as to their use from December 31, 1983 (*DHSS*, 1983(8), para. 6). Annex B to the Circular provides further guidance on how the Secretary of State will define restriction of liberty for the purpose of the regulations. (*DHSS*, 1983).

Before any child can be kept in secure accommodation the criteria set out above in section 21A(1) must first be satisfied. The regulations provide that no child under ten years of age can be confined unless the local authority first obtains the consent of the Secretary of State (reg. 4). However, in certain exceptional cases the statutory criteria do not apply, and in these cases the regulations provide the relevant criteria. Thus, where a child has been committed to the care of a local authority while on remand or following committal for trial (C.Y.P.A. 1969, s.23) *and*: (a) has either been charged with or convicted of an offence imprisonable in the case of a person aged 21 or over for 14 years or more; or (b) has been charged with or convicted of an offence of violence, or previously convicted of an offence of violence *and* if in either case it appears that he needs to be kept in secure accommodation either because he is likely to abscond, or to injure himself or other people if kept anywhere else, then the requirements of section 21A(1) do not apply. (reg. 7). Where any child in the care of a local authority is placed in secure accommodation which is not managed by his care authority the local authority which manages that accommodation is under a duty to inform the care authority within 24 hours of placement. (reg. 9.)

The Regulations specify 72 hours as the maximum period beyond which a child in the care of a local authority may not be kept in secure accommodation without the authority of a juvenile court. It should be noted that this period may be of 72 hours consecutively or an aggregate of that number in any consecutive period of 28 days. Where it is intended to apply to the juvenile court for authority to keep the child in secure accommodation for a longer period then the parents or guardian of the child must be informed as soon as possible (reg. 15), and this will facilitate an early application for legal aid on the child's behalf. In addition the care authority should ensure that the child's independent visitor, if one has been appointed, is similarly informed (reg. 15). It is provided that the maximum period for which a juvenile court may authorise a child to be kept in secure accommodation is three months (reg. 8–12) but the statute provides that this power of authorisation cannot be exercised unless the child has either applied for and been given or refused legal aid, or having been given the opportunity has failed to apply the Child Care Act 1980, s.21A(6). The regulations allow for the juvenile court to authorise a further period in secure accommodation not exceeding six months. (reg. 9–13). The statute provides that in the event of a juvenile court adjourning its consideration of an application, an interim order may be made and the child placed in approved secure accommodation or in a Youth Treatment Centre for the duration of the adjournment (s.21A(4) and 4. *DHSS*, 1983(8) para. 33).

The Regulations make provision for, and the DHSS stresses that great importance attaches to, the review of the cases of children being kept in secure accommodation (regs. 16 and 17). Regulation 11 requires the care authority of any child in care placed in secure accommodation to ensure that his case is reviewed at intervals not exceeding three months and to appoint at least two persons to undertake this function. When so appointed their duties are to satisfy themselves in respect of each case that the criteria for keeping the child in secure accommodation continue to apply and the placement continues to be appropriate for the child at that stage, and in doing so they must have regard to the future requirements of the child (reg. 16). The persons undertaking the review must further ascertain and take into account the views of the child, his parent or guardian if practicable, any other persons who have had the care of the child, the child's independent visitor, if one has been appointed, and the managing authority if different from the child's care authority. These parties must all be informed of the outcome of the review (reg. 15). Regulation 13–18 requires each local authority responsible for the management of secure accommodation to keep records giving:

(a) the name, date of birth, sex of the child;
(b) details of the care order or other statutory provision under which the child is in the community home and particulars of any other local authority involved with the placement of the child;
(c) the date, time and reason for the placement, the name of the officer authorising placement, and where the child was living before placement;
(d) persons informed, court orders made and reviews undertaken in respect of each child;
(e) the date and time of the child's discharge from secure accommodation and his subsequent residence.

These records must be available for inspection by the Secretary of State, and the Secretary of State can require copies to be forwarded to him at any time. (reg. 18).

The 1983 Regulations revoke regulations 11 to 14 of the Community Homes Regulations 1972 which are otherwise left intact. The 1983 regulations can be welcomed on several counts for not only do they provide children deprived of their liberty for periods in excess of 72 hours with the right of access to the courts, but the conditions under which they can be so deprived in the first place, and can continue to be so deprived by the courts are considerably tighter than those initially proposed by the Government at the report stage of the Criminal Justice Bill. Thus, the possible criteria had included simple absconding, and likelihood of damage to or taking of another person's property, which would have allowed a child to be locked up simply for running away from an unsuitable or unhappy placement in a community home, or because there was a risk that the child might have been about to commit a minor offence. This seemed extraordinary especially since the DHSS's own working party had rejected absconding as a criterion for locking up children (*DHSS*, 1981). Thus, as it pointed out, "absconding and other extremes of behaviour may well be due to anxiety about domestic circumstances or unhappiness in current placement. It is not sufficient for youngsters to be placed in security and deprived of their liberty simply because they abscond or because a more suitable environment with a high staff ratio and specialist advice is not available elsewhere." (*DHSS*, 1981). It would seem from the wording of the statute and the regulations that the Government took some notice of these and similar findings, it remains however to be seen whether these words are interpreted in the right spirit by local authorities and juvenile courts alike.

Compliance with the regulations

The primary duty of complying with the regulations in each case lies with the responsible body for each community home but while these bodies may give guidance as to the implementation of the regulations, they must rely on the person in charge of the home for the day to day conduct of the home. As far as inspections are concerned, usually carried out by the DHSS under the terms of section 74 of the Child Care Act 1980 (see below, p. 74), the person in charge of the home is under a duty to give to an inspector such information as he may require about the home, its state and management, the children and their treatment, and to give access to any written records kept in relation to the home.

III. *Regulation of Voluntary Homes*

The Secretary of State also has power under the 1980 Act to make regulations as to the conduct of voluntary homes (s.60). The governing regulations at the present time are the Administration of Children's Homes Regulations 1951. Before the passing of the Community Homes Regulation 1972, the 1951 Regulations also applied to homes run by the local authority but since nearly all local authority homes are now community homes, the 1951 Regulations chiefly apply to voluntary homes.

The regulations follow the general principle laid down in the Act, in providing that the body responsible for running the home should make arrangements to ensure that it is conducted in such a manner and on such principles as are calculated to secure the well-being of the children in the house. The body responsible for running the home has the power to appoint the person in charge, (though the Secretary of State must be notified of any change), and also to ensure that the home is visited at least once a month by someone who must be satisfied that the home is being run in accordance with the principles set out above. This person must report to the responsible body upon his visit and the details of the visit must be entered in the home's record book.

Day-to-day care of children

The regulations make detailed provision as to the arrangements to be made for the medical and dental care of the children, the keeping of medical records, and the standard of cleanliness and hygiene to be observed in the home (regs. 5 and 6). The person in charge of the home is under a duty to notify the local authority and the child's parent or guardian in those circumstances where a child dies or suffers serious injury or illness of where infectious illness has broken out in the home.

As far as the safety of children is concerned, the responsible body is directed to consult the fire authority as to fire precautions in the home, and to make arrangements to secure by means of fire drills and practices that the staff in the home and as far as is practicable the children are well versed in the procedure for saving life in the case of fire (regs. 8 and 9).

The person in charge is also expected to ensure that there are facilities available for parents or guardians to visit children in the home and to communicate with them. The Secretary of State can also ask for information on such facilities or issue direction as to their provision.

Freedom of religion

As far as the religious well-being of children in these homes in concerned, the responsible body is under a duty to secure that each child attends such religious services and receives religious instruction as is appropriate to the religious pursuasion to which he belongs, and is practicable in the circumstances. At first sight therefore it would appear that these regulations impose more stringent requirements than do the 1972 Regulations, which merely provide for the affording of the *opportunity*. Even under the 1951 Regulations however, the duty is limited to what is practicable in the circumstances of the case.

Control of children

The 1951 Regulations make much more detailed provision as to the control of children in the home than do the Community Homes Regulations 1972. The 1951 Regulations contain specific directions on corporal punishment whereas the 1972 Regulations left much to the discretion of the responsible body subject to prior local authority approval. The DHSS commented in 1972 that there had been a decline in the use of corporal punishment and expressed the hope that it would be phased out generally, but have done little to ensure that this occurs (see above, p. 65). The staff in voluntary homes are, therefore, able to inflict corporal punishment provided certain conditions are satisfied (reg. 11). Thus punishment may only be administered by the person in charge of the home or his deputy, if he is ill or away, to girls under the age of 10, or boys under the age of 16. In the case of a child under 10, corporal punishment can only be administered by smacking on the hands with a bare hand, and in the case of boys between 10 and 16, they may receive up to six strokes of the cane upon their clothed posteriors. It is further provided that no caning should be administered in the presence of another child, and that where a child has any physical or mental disability, punishment should only be given where the medical officer has sanctioned such a measure. Where any punishment is administered the regulations require details of that punishment to be entered in a book kept specifically for that purpose. There are no provisions in the 1951 Regulations for locking children up or for any form of secure accommodation to be used within voluntary homes.

Compliance with the regulations

The primary duty for ensuring compliance rests with the organisation running the home, but the person in charge is clearly the one with immediate responsibility. In particular, the regulations specifically provide that it is he who must compile the various records recognised by the regulations including registers of children in the home, a record book recording events of importance in the home, and records of food provided, fire precautions taken, and fire practices and drills held in the home. He is further responsible for the custody of the medical record of each child in the home, which should always be available to the medical officer. Should anyone contravene or fail to comply with any of the regulations or any requirements or directions issued thereunder, he will be guilty of an offence and liable on summary conviction to a fine not exceeding £500.

Official visiting of children in voluntary homes

In addition to the general powers of entry and inspection possessed by the DHSS (see below, p. 74) the 1980 Act imposes a duty on local authorities to cause children in voluntary homes in their area to be visited *in the interests of their well-being*. Any person authorised to carry out such visits by the local authority, may exercise powers of entry and inspection on production of some duly authenticated document. Visits may be conducted by representatives of a local authority in a home outside the area of that local authority, where children in their care have for various reasons had to be accommodated at a distance. Where the voluntary home is found to be in breach of any of the regulations, the Secretary of State has power under the 1980 Act to cancel the home's registration (s.57).

IV. *Regulation of Private Children's Homes*

Pursuant to the implementation of the Children's Homes Act 1982, the Secretary of State now has power to make regulations as to the conduct of homes registered in accordance with the provisions of that Act. Before the passage of that Act, although the DHSS had powers of entry and inspection (see below, p. 74) the Secretary of State had no power upon discovery or proof of unsatisfactory conditions following such inspections, to require the home to institute changes of any sort, to require the removal of children (save under C.Y.P.A. 1969, s.28—place of safety provisions) or to prevent further admissions.

The 1982 Act provides for the making of regulations so closely resembling those relating to voluntary homes that it is possible that the Administration of Children's Homes Regulations 1951 may simply be extended to apply to privately run homes. Thus, the statute provides that regulations may be made concerning the medical, psychiatric and dental welfare of children; limiting the number of children to be accommodated in any home, facilitating their upbringing in the religious pursuasion to which they adhere, requiring notice of any change of appointment of the person running the home, and imposing requirements as to the keeping of records in respect of the children. The local authority which registers the home is given powers of entry and inspection, which extend not only to the premises, but also to the children and to any records kept in relation to the home. Anyone obstructing an officer of the responsible authority in the exercise of his functions will be guilty of an offence and liable on summary conviction to a fine not exceeding £500. In addition, any refusal to allow an officer to enter shall be deemed for the purposes of issuing warrants under section 40 of the Children and Young Persons Act 1933, to be a reasonable cause to suspect that a child in the home is being neglected in a manner likely to cause him unnecessary suffering or injury to health. If the local authority which registered the home has reason to believe that it is not being carried on in accordance with these regulations, or with any other requirements, it can cancel the home's registration. This can occur either at the time of the annual review of registration or at any other time.

V. *General Provisions affecting all Children's Residential Homes*

The Child Care Act 1980 provides the Secretary of State with powers to authorise the inspection of all premises where children in care are accommodated and of the children themselves except where any such home is the responsibility of another Government department. An example of such an exception would be special residential schools for maladjusted children which are subject instead to inspection by Her Majesty's Inspector of Schools, being the responsibility of the Department of Education and Science (s.74).

These powers of inspection are exercised on behalf of the Secretary of State, normally by officers of the Children's Department of the DHSS although exceptionally officer of a local authority may conduct inspections provided that authority consents. Anyone authorised to conduct an inspection has a right to enter any premises covered by the Act on production of some duly authenticated document proving his right of entry. Obstructing the exercise of this power of entry may render an offender liable to summary prosecution and, if convicted, a fine. In addition, refusal to allow entry will be deemed to be a reasonable cause to suspect that a child is being neglected in a manner likely to cause him unnecessary suffering or injury to health and will thus constitute grounds for the issuing of a warrant under section 40 of the Children and Young Persons Act 1933 (s.75).

Where the Secretary of State has reason to be concerned about the way in which matters connected with children's care are being administered, he has, since 1975, had the power under the statute to cause an inquiry to be held, which upon his direction may be held in private. The power to order such inquiries was expected to be used extremely sparingly. There have in fact been several inquiries into child abuse cases. A committee of inquiry is empowered to *subpoena* witnesses, take evidence on oath, and require the production of documents (s.76). Local Authorities and Juvenile Courts are placed under a duty to give the Secretary of State such particulars as he may require as to the exercise by them of their powers and duties under the child care legislation, to enable him to report fully to Parliament (s.79). A similar provision relates to voluntary organisations to enable details of the performance of their functions to be included in any such report.

Finally, to enable the Secretary of State to discharge his functions more efficiently, the 1980 Act provided for the continued existence of the Advisory Council on Child Care. However, this body which in its time had produced some very useful reports (see for example "Care and Treatment in a Planned Environment," *DHSS, A.C.C.* 1971) was finally abolished by section 27 of the Health and Social Services and Social Security Adjudications Act 1983.

VI. *Regulation of other Residential Accommodation for Children*

(a) Physically handicapped children

The quality of residential care in special boarding schools or long-stay hospitals for children with a physical handicap has only

rarely exercised the minds of those Committees which have investigated the life of children in care. In consequence, perhaps, residential care for these groups has not been subject to the same legal
control or regulation as other forms of care. Thus, for example,
the Curtis Committee (1946) thought that the care of physically
handicapped children living away from home was largely outside
their scope and so did not consider it. Partly, this was because
these children were often not "in care" in the way in which
orphans or those compulsorily removed from home were, and
partly because they were being looked after in "acceptable" establishments, either in special boarding schools or receiving necessary
treatment in long-stay hospitals.

Regulation of special boarding schools

The Curtis Committee, while broadly in favour of the principle
of extending special boarding school education for those with
physical handicaps, was of the opinion that their care should also
fall within the remit of Ministry of Education. Essentially, this
remains the system of control even today.

Special boarding schools for handicapped children like other
schools have to be registered under the Education Act 1944 and in
order to achieve registration they must comply with the conditions
laid down in the Handicapped Pupils and Special Schools Regulations 1959, and amendments made in 1980, and any conditions laid
down in further regulations issued under section 12 of the Education Act 1981. Thus, they must meet minimum requirements as
to staffing levels and qualifications and the condition of the premises to be used and the facilities offered. These schools are subject
to the inspection powers of the Department of Education and Science, undertaken on behalf of the Secretary of State by Her Majesty's Inspectors of Schools. The Inspectors have the right of entry
to all schools under the 1944 Act and are responsible for inspecting
both the educational and boarding facilities. Where the Inspectors
find anything to cause concern, they have the power to make
recommendations for improvements, and where the body fails to
take notice of such a recommendation, the Secretary of State may
serve a notice of complaint. This requires the responsible body to
carry out the recommendations within a certain period of time, the
penalty for failure being cancellation of the school's registration.
Little guidance, however, has been given on the standards of care

to be exercised on the residential side. It has been suggested that the DHSS and the Department of Education and Science should examine how far the principle of dual registration, *i.e.* as a home and as a special school, which applies to residential educational facilities for mentally handicapped children, could be extended to residential educational establishments for the physically handicapped (*Shearer*, 1980). This is more especially the case in the light of the Warnock Committee's recommendation that each school should have a deputy-head who would be in charge of residential care. (*Warnock Report*, 1978).

Regulation of long-stay hospitals

The monitoring of standards of care of physically handicapped children in long-stay hospitals was, after the establishment of the National Health Service, the responsibility of hospital management committees. They were subject to the control in turn of the regional hospital boards and ultimately the Minister of Health had overall responsibility (see *Oswin*, 1978). No inspectorate similar to those existing for children in care and for those in special boarding schools exists for those handicapped children in long-stay hospitals, who are not technically "in care." They do not even have the protection afforded to children in care by virtue of the six-monthly review (see above, pp. 34 and 54). Although the first draft of the scheme for the National Health Service had in fact envisaged the establishment of a health inspectorate responsible for hospital care, the nearest anyone ever got to this was when Richard Crossman announced his intention of adopting such a system following the publication of the Report on Ely Hospital (1969). Feeling within the health service and amongst civil servants ran so high, however, that he was forced to be content with a professional scrutiny or advisory service, though he did insist that this be independent of the DHSS (*Crossman*, 1977). Thus, the Hospital (later Health) Advisory Service was born. In its first year it concentrated on a survey of the country's mental handicap hospitals but its remit was later extended to cover the whole range of health and social service provision for all long-stay groups. Indeed in 1972, the Advisory service reported that hospital children can live in conditions which fall far short of the standards of child care expected in other residential accommodation (*National Health Service* 1973).

Shearer (1980) states that the Hospital Advisory Service has also shown that because of over-provision of paediatric beds, children are kept in hospital or even admitted for social reasons and tend to become "long-stay" without anyone really noticing, when they do not even need the services provided by a hospital (see also *DHSS*, 1970 and *Oswin*, 1978). Clearly, such children should be brought within the regulating scope of the ordinary child care legislation even though the majority are not in the care of the local authority. Shearer (1980) states that what is needed for these children is a ministerial directive along the following lines:

(a) All children living for more than four months in a non-psychiatric hospital will be reviewed by a joint health, social services and education team within 12 months, and plans made for their future.

(b) Only those who can be shown to need active medical treatment will remain in hospital. The others will be found new homes within the normal range of provision for children away from their family within one year.

(c) Those who do remain in hospital will live in special units jointly staffed by residential child care workers and nurses under the overall charge of a child care worker, and be reviewed *monthly* by a multi-disciplinary team including medical, nursing social services and educational staff to plan for their future outside the unit.

Although, as Shearer comments, this programme is only a modest one, until implementation of directives along these lines, the authorities concerned would be well advised for the sake of the children to adopt such a programme on a voluntary basis.

(b) Children in legal custody

(i) *In community homes*

Some children who are being held in custody pending investigation of or prosecution for the commission of a criminal offence, may be remanded into the care of the local authority, which will then have to accommodate them in a community home (C.Y.P.A. 1969, s.23(1)). A child so placed will be subject to the same controls as children in these homes who are in the care of the local authority under other provisions (see above, p. 28). Similarly, those children who have been ordered to be detained by a local authority following conviction on indictment for certain serious crimes, and who are housed in a community home, are also subject to all the conditions laid down in the Community Homes Regulations 1972 (C.Y.P.A. 1933, s.53, C.Y.P.A. 1969, s.30), and the Secure Accommodation Regulations 1983 (C.C.A. 1980, s.17 and C.C.A. 1980, s.21A inserted by C.J.A. 1982, s.25).

(ii) *In remand centres*

Where the court has issued a certificate of unruly character (see p. 55), and provided a remand centre place is available, the child will be committed to the centre (C.Y.P.A. 1969, s.23(2)) and while there will be subject to its rules and to the provisions of the Prison Act 1952 (as amended). Since section 65 of the Criminal Justice Act 1967 outlawed corporal punishment in any institutions to which the 1952 Act applies, it is unlawful to administer corporal punishment to children held in these establishments. Any child removed from a community home to a remand centre under section 23(3) of the Children and Young Persons Act 1969 will be subject to the same regulation.

(iii) *In prisons*

Children, who for one reason or another find themselves in the Young Persons wing of a prison, either pursuant to the issue of a certificate of unruly character or on conviction where there are no places available in youth custody centres, will be subject to the provision of the Prison Act 1952 as amended. Corporal punishment is thus illegal, and any complaints about treatment can be made to the Board of Prison Visitors.

(iii) *In detention centres*

The Detention Centre Rules 1983 contain those provisions regulating care in these establishments with an obvious concentration on matters concerning discipline and control. Indeed, the regimen implied by the very detailed rules is almost military in character.

Day-to-day care. There are provisions regulating search of inmates, and medical examination upon reception at the centre and the centre's Medical Officer has wide ranging responsibilities for the supervision of such matters as hygiene, diet and the consumption of drink and tobacco. The Medical Officer must also visit any inmate confined to a detention room and must be informed of the use of mechanical restraints upon any detaineee and be given the opportunity to make recommendations regarding their use.

Contact with the detainee's family is encouraged to the extent deemed desirable in his best interests, and he is to be encouraged and assisted to maintain or establish such relations with persons or agencies outside the Centre as may promote his social rehabilitation. There are detailed provisions regarding the receipt of letters and visits from friends and family, both of which may be subject to supervision and may be deferred as a disciplinary measure, but visits for special purposes—for example by the police officer or legal representative are *not* liable to deferrment.

Where the detainee is under 16, arrangements must be made for his full-time education, and if over 16, can be made for part-time education. Detainees may, if over 16, be employed for a working week of 44 hours, but at least one hour a day must be devoted to physical training or organised games and those periods are included as part of the working week. Exemption from work or physical training can be given by the Medical Officer who also has to certify any detainee as being fit for the type of work allotted to him.

Freedom of religion. Upon reception, every inmate's religious denomination must be recorded and, where this is other than Church of England, the detainee must be informed of his right to request at the centre the attendance of a minister of his denomination, so far as this is practicable. Work on Sundays, or the recognised days of religious observance of other religions, is to be avoided, and arrangements must be made for visits by a minister where a detainee is sick or dying.

Control. Control of discipline within the centres is the primary responsibility of the Warden, or his deputy or delegate in his absence. Where an offence against discipline by a detainee is reported, he may be kept separate and apart from other inmates, but before he is dealt with he must be informed of the offence for which he has been reported, and be given a proper opportunity of hearing the facts alleged against him and of presenting his case. Where the offence is proved, he may be punished under the powers given to the Warden, or under those given to the Board of Visitors. Punishment can include disqualification from recreational activities, the imposition of extra fatigues, removal to a detention room, withdrawal of privileges, and forfeiture of remission of up to seven days, all of which can be imposed by the Warden. Where the Warden thinks it expedient the case can be referred to the Board of Visitors who have the same powers of punishment but for longer periods. The 1952 Rules also provided for confinement to a detention room and a restricted diet by way of punishment but the Home Office has indicated (*Home Office*, 1971) that rules would be laid before Parliament to provide for the abolition of dietary punishment and confinement, in accordance with the recommendations made by the *Advisory Council on the Penal System* (1971). Where the detainee has been of good conduct the rules provide for the remission of the detention centre order, which can now be up to one-half of the original sentence.

Compliance with the regulations. Responsibility for ensuring compliance rests initially with the Warden who is supposed to exercise a close and constant personal supervision of the whole centre. Any complaints by detainees must be recorded and be put forward to be dealt with by the body to whom the complaint was addressed, be this the Warden or the Board of Visitors. The Board of Visitors is required by the rules to meet at the centre at least once a month to discharge its functions and it must frequently visit and inspect the centre and make such recommendations to the Secretary of State as it thinks fit. At the end of each year they must also make an annual report to him with regard to all or any of the matters referred to in the Rules, including advice and suggestions on any matters arising to do with the Centre.

(v) *Children in youth custody centres*

Following the change over to youth custody sentences, from Borstal training, which took effect in May 1983, new rules governing the regulation of such centres were issued by the Secretary of State. The Youth Custody Centre Rules 1983 are very similar in substance to the Prison and Borstal Rules 1964. Given that the youth custody centres have taken on the premises, staff and in reality the functions of borstals, it was unlikely that the rules would be very different (*Home Office, Welsh Office, DHSS*, 1980). The new rules specifically provide that "the aims of a youth custody centre shall be to provide work, training and instruction of a kind that will assist offenders to acquire or develop personal resources, interests and skills; to encourage offenders to exercise self-discipline and accept responsibility; to foster their links with the outside community; and to help them with their return to the community in co-operation with the services responsible for supervision" (r.3). Youth custody centre inmates are to be occupied according to individual assessment and development in work, training, education and physical education for up to 40 hours a week or eight hours a day, and will be paid for any work done (r.34). There is to be at least 15 hours of education and vocational training for those of compulsory school age and arrangements made for appropriate education of those "illiterate or backward" (r.37(1) and (2)). Women under 21 detained in youth custody centres instead of prison are to have "reasonable facilities" if they wish to improve their education (r.37(3)). There is to be physical education within the working week as well as at weekends and during evenings (r.38). Order and discipline are to be maintained " . . . with no more restriction than is required in the interests of security and well-ordered community life" (r.41(1)). The exact length of a youth custody sentence is fixed by the court: thus any breaches of centre discipline can only lead to a reduction of any remission for good behaviour. The Youth Custody Centre's Board of Visitors is under similar duties to visit, hear complaints and make reports as the Board of Visitors for Detention Centres (see above, p. 81).

(ii) *Children in intermediate treatment residential facilities*

This group of children is anomalous in the sense that they are not strictly speaking being detained in legal custody nor are they in the care of the local authority, though many are undergoing treatment pursuant to an order following their conviction for a criminal offence. The power and duty to provide intermediate treatment facilities derives from section 12(2) and (3), (3A–3C) of the Children and Young Persons Act 1969 as amended by the Criminal Justice Act 1982, under which as part of either a "discretionary" or "stipulated" intermediate treatment requirement (see above, p. 12 and below, pp. 111–113) included in a supervision order made in criminal proceedings, a supervised person could be directed to live for a period or periods of up to 90 days at a specified place, or such shorter period as the supervisor, (s.12(3)) or the court (s.12(3)(e)) shall direct, (C.Y.P.A. 1969, s.12 as amended). The specified place can be an intermediate treatment residential centre. The DHSS states that a variety of residential centres is provided by different agencies (*DHSS*, 1977) and that their use should normally form part of a comprehensive intermediate treatment programme for the children concerned. Some special 90-day intermediate treatment centres have been established and some authorities use community homes with education on the premises for this purpose. Other centres operate for shorter periods, many providing weekend residential facilities or short weekly courses.

The aim of such residential centres is, according to the DHSS, to provide experiences which it is not possible to provide in a community based scheme, experiences shared between staff and children (*DHSS*, 1977). Contact with the child's family is positively encouraged.

Control of children undergoing such treatment is in the hands of staff running the centre but the supervisor is supposed to keep in close contact with the staff and also with the child (*DHSS*, 1972). The DHSS suggests that frequent and regular reviews of the child's progress should be held (*DHSS*, 1977) and, where the child commits any breaches of discipline and the treatment order was imposed following conviction for a criminal offence, he may be taken back to court and dealt with by means of a fine or attendance centre order (Criminal Law Act 1977, s.37 and see below, p. 113) or a care order may be substituted (C.Y.P.A. 1969, s.15). There are no specialised rules or regulations governing the conduct of centres at which intermediate treatment courses may be run but guidance as to the scope, organisation and regulation of these facilities issues from time to time from the DHSS (see *DHSS*, 1972 and 1977). The most recent of these states that the longer stay intermediate treatment centres are more appropriate as a means of reorientation leading into further community-based work. The emphasis, therefore, is much more on treatment rather than on punishment (*DHSS*, 1977), though, as has been indicated elsewhere, the efficacy of such treatment has yet to be proved to the satisfaction of either social workers or courts, (below, p. 115).

4. Maintenance of Children in Residential Care

I. *Contributions towards Maintenance*

A. Children in care of local authority

1. Under Child Care Act 1980, s.2 or by virtue of a care order

General. The provisions described in this section apply wherever the child has been received into care under section 2 of the Child Care Act 1980 or is the subject of a care order made under the Children and Young Persons Act 1969, regardless of the type of accommodation in which he may have been placed. Thus, contributions will be payable whether the child has been placed by the local authority in a local authority community home, a controlled or assisted community home, a voluntary home, a private children's home, a hospital ward, or special school or whether he has been boarded out. (As to which see *Hoggett*, 1981).

Liability. Where a child has been received into care or is the subject of a care order, and is under 16 years of age, his mother and father may be liable to make contributions to the local authority in respect of his maintenance, and where he is over 16, the child himself may be liable to make such contributions (C.C.A. 1980, s.45(1), as amended by H. & S.S. & S.S.A.A. 1983, s.19). The effect of the most recent changes is that where the child is under 16, a parent will be liable to make contributions unless he is in receipt of benefits under the Supplementary Benefits Act 1976 or in receipt of family income supplement. Once the child attains the age of 16 however the parent ceases to be liable, and liability falls upon the child himself whether *or not* he is in full-time work. So if the child is in receipt of supplementary benefit, the local authority may seek a contribution from him. Where the child is illegitimate, it is the mother alone who is liable in the first instance but arrangements can be made for the local authority to receive any payments made under an affiliation order (s.49(2)) and if no steps have ever been taken to obtain such an order, the authority may itself initiate proceedings (C.C.A. 1980, s.50). Where a contribution order has been made it is suspended for such periods as the child is allowed by the local authority to be under the charge or control of his parent or guardian (s.45(3)) or upon receipt by the local authority of a notice of intention to apply for adoption of the child (Adoption Act 1958 s.36(2)).

Amount of contribution. The 1980 Act, as amended by the H. & S.S. & S.S.A.A. 1983, provides that the amount of a contribution shall be such amount as may be specified in a notice in writing (a "contribution notice") served on the liable person by the local authority and agreed by him or, in default of agreement, as shall be determined by the court in proceedings for, or for variation of, a contribution order (s.46(1)). The maximum contribution which may be specified in a contribution notice shall be not greater than the weekly amount which in the opinion of the local authority, they would normally be prepared to pay if a child of the same age were boarded out by them. Subject to that limitation the amount may either be a standard contribution determined by the local authority for all children in their care, or such other amount as the local authority consider reasonable in the circumstances. Since the amounts paid out by local authorities in fostering allowances are considerably less than the amount required to accommodate a child in a residential home, nothing approaching the full costs of keeping a child in a residential care will ever be recovered from the parents. What research there is on the income levels of parents whose children are in the care of the local authority shows that they are by and large amongst the lowest income groups (*Packman,* 1968, *Holman,* 1980, *S.S.R.I.U.,* 1980). Many are unemployed or when employed earn markedly less than the national average wage. The issue of contributions may, therefore, be a difficult one to sort out and many social workers feel that attempts to force it may well jeopardise the work they may be doing with the families.

As to the charges actually suggested by local authorities some, for example, Wandsworth, operate a basic flat rate contribution system but the majority of authorities conduct a means test on parental incomes (*Wandsworth*, 1980). Since many parents are in the lower income groups such tests often result in a "nil" assessment for contributions, and the statute does not impose a duty to collect from parents, merely a discretion so to do. The 1983 Act further allows the local authority the discretion at any time to withdraw a contribution notice (without prejudice to their power to serve another) or not to serve one at all in any case where in the circumstances they consider it unreasonable to require contributions (C.C.A. 1980, s.46, as amended by H. & S.S. & S.S.A.A. 1983, s.19). Similarly, if the local authority should decide to apply to the court for a contribution order, the court could in its discretion make a "nil" order.

Contribution orders. Where the local authority and the liable contributor have failed to agree as to the amount of any contribution or the contributor has defaulted, an application may be made to the local magistrates' court for a contribution order which the court may make, provided certain conditions are satisfied. An order cannot be made unless either the care authority has specified an amount in a contribution notice served on the liable person (which has not been withdrawn), and the liable person has not within one month agreed with the local authority on the amount of his contribution, or the contributor has defaulted in making *two* or more contributions of an amount agreed with the local authority at any time (C.C.A. 1980, s.47(1), as amended by H. & S.S. & S.S.A.A., 1983, s.19). It has been suggested (*Home Office*, 1970) that where the care authority is not the authority to which contributions are payable (see below, p. 87 and s.53) the care authority should send the other authority a copy of the notice and should notify the authority of any agreement or failure to agree. In the alternative it is suggested that the care authority might arrange for the other authority to give notice on its behalf, in which case the notice should state that it is given on behalf of the care authority.

In proceedings for a contribution order the court cannot order a contributor to pay a contribution greater than the amount specified in the contribution notice (C.C.A. 1980, s.47(2), as amended by H. & S.S. & S.S.A.A. 1983, s.19). Thus, where the authority applying for the order is not the care authority, it must inform the court of the amount proposed by the care authority. The court may decide to confirm the amount by order, or having regard to the contributor's means, it can make such lesser order as it thinks fit. Similarly, in any proceedings for the variation of a contribution order the care authority must specify to the court the amount which it proposes, and the amount of any order must be no greater than that specified (s.48(2)). The form of the contribution order can be found in Form 54 in Schedule 2 to the Magistrates' Courts' (Children and Young Persons) Rules 1970. Proceedings may also be taken against persons residing in Scotland or Northern Ireland (s.55).

Duration of orders. A contribution order remains in force for so long as the child is in the care of the local authority concerned (s.47(3)) but will not in any event extend beyond the date when the child reaches the age of 16 (s.45(4)).

Enforcement. Contribution orders are enforceable by means of proceedings for attachment of earnings, distress, and where there is wilful refusal or culpable neglect to pay and attachment of earnings is deemed to be an inappropriate method of enforcement, the court may commit the offending contributor to prison (s.47(4)).

Default on contributions or orders. Arrears of payment can be recovered by the local authority where a parent has defaulted on payment of agreed contributions (s.51) by means of proceedings for an arrears order. The arrears order may require the contributor to pay such weekly sum for such period as the court having regard to his means thinks fit. The aggregate of payments which may be ordered must not exceed the aggregate, which would have been payable under a contribution order in respect of the period of default, or, if it exceeds three months, the last three months as well as any period equal to the time during which the default continued after the making of the application for the arrears order.

Where any arrears have arisen pursuant to the obtaining of a contribution order, the local authority in whose area the contributor is residing (which need not be the care authority) can receive, and if necessary enforce, payment of any arrears, even though the arrears did not accrue when the liable contributor was resident in the area (s.54(1)).

Transmission of contributions as between local authorities. If contributions or arrears are received by a local authority and another authority is responsible for the maintenance of the child, the first authority is under a duty to pay over the amounts received subject to any such deductions in respect of services rendered by that authority as may be agreed (s.53).

Affiliation orders. Where a child is in the care of a local authority, other than under an interim order, the magistrates' court may order payments under an affiliation order for the child's maintenance which is already in force to be made to the local authority entitled to receive contributions (s.50(4)). Should the child cease to be in the care of the local authority or, while remaining in care is allowed to be under the charge or control of a parent or guardian, relative or friend, the affiliation order ceases to be operative (s.49(6)). The mother or the person with custody, however, can then apply to have the order revived.

If there is no affiliation order in force in respect of an illegitimate child, the Act allows the local authority to apply for such an order. Application for an order should be made by the local authority within three years of the date when the child was received into care or the care order came into force. The Act further provides that if an order is granted but later ceases if the child leaves care, the local authority can later seek revival of the affiliation order should the child subsequently return to care (s.50(5)). Under the provisions of the Affiliation Proceedings (Amendment) Act 1972, an affiliation order may be made by the court without the local authority having to rely on the mother to give evidence. Appeals against the making of an affiliation order or its amount lie to the Crown Court.

Appeals against contribution, arrears and transfer orders. Appeals lie to the Crown Court from the Magistrates' Court in respect of contribution orders and arrears orders, by the liable contributor or in the case of an order transferring affiliation payments to the local authority, by the person (usually the mother) who would otherwise be entitled to the payments. The collection of parental contributions and the taking of proceedings for contribution orders is by no means uniform practice across the country. The reasons for this are that the amounts collected or ordered are often small, and the administrative, legal and social work costs are, as Morgan (1981) points out disproportionately high compared with the amount collected. Enquiries made of three large social services departments in the North-West of England and research conducted by Morgan (1981) in Leicestershire confirmed that such exercises are not cost-effective. The purpose behind them is, as Morgan suggests, a reinforcement of family responsibility, which has its roots in the poor law. Official comment on the practice of collecting contributions and taking proceedings for contribution orders has been scant (*Layfield*, 1974, *Recommendations on Local Government Finance*, 1977) and the only official guidelines (*Home Office*, 1970) give no hint as to the thinking of central government on this delicate issue. Since the statutory provisions seem to leave discretion with the local authority, it is up to each department to decide its own policy. Few go the way of Wandsworth, and most opt for a case by case merits approach in respect of both agreed contributions and contribution orders.

2. Children committed into the care of the local authority

(a) *Under guardianship legislation*

Liability. Where a child has been committed to the care of a local authority pursuant to a custody application under section 9 of the Guardianship of Minors Act 1971, the court is given the power by section 2(2)(*b*) of the Guardianship Act 1973 to require either parent to pay over to the authority, or to the child himself, such periodical payments and for such term as may be specified in the order. These maintenance payments need only be paid to the local authority while the child continues in its care, (Guardianship Act 1973, s.2(3)), but the local authority, the child himself if over 16, or the party liable to make such payments, may apply for variation or revocation of a periodical payments order (G.A. 1973, s.4(3A)).

Duration. An order for periodical payments made under these provisions will last until the child's 17th birthday unless the court specifies a later date, and shall not in any event extend beyond the child's reaching the age of 18, unless the child is continuing in full-time education or there are special circumstances (G.A. 1973, s.2(3B)). When making an order the court is directed to have regard to all the circumstances of the case and to the guidelines laid down in section 12A of the Guardianship of Minors Act 1971 relating to such matters as parents' income, earning capacity and their financial needs and responsibilities as well as the child's financial needs and any physical or mental disabilities.

(b) *Under the adoption and foster care legislation*

Where, for whatever reason, the court refuses an application for an adoption order, in respect of a child previously in care, and that child is returned to the local authority's care then any arrangements made earlier regarding contributions can be revived either by agreement or if necessary by court order (Adoption Act 1958, s.36(2)).

The Children Act 1975 introduced new powers for the court on refusal of an adoption application, which apply to all cases, whether or not the original placement was done by an agency (s.17). This includes the power to commit the child to the care of a specified local authority, and to make an order requiring either parent to pay to that authority such weekly or other periodical sum towards the maintenance of the child as the court thinks reasonable (s.17(2)). The provisions of the Guardianship Act 1973 relating to duration, powers of variation and revocation of orders apply also in relation to these orders (s.17(3)).

A child removed from a private foster placement by a local authority pursuant to a place of safety order granted under the Foster Children Act 1980 may be received into care as if under section 2 of the Child Care Act 1980, despite the fact that no section 2 grounds are established. The provisions of the Child Care Act 1980 relating to contributions and orders therefore apply to this very small group of children (F.C.A. 1980, s.12).

(c) *Under matrimonial legislation*

Similar orders to those made under the guardianship legislation can also be made in those situations where the court is approached because of the breakdown of the parents' marriage. In both magistrates' domestic proceedings and in divorce courts the court may make an order committing a child into the care of the local authority.

(i) *Magistrates' Court orders.* Where a committal to care order is made under section 11(4) of the 1978 Act the court may make a further order requiring a party to the marriage in question to make to that authority or to the child himself such periodical payments in accordance with the guidelines laid down in section 3, and for such term as may be specified in the order.

DURATION. The provisions as to duration of orders for periodical payments are the same as those made where custody of the child is given to the parent (s.11(6)). The order can extend in the first instance to the age of 17 though it can be extended to 18, and beyond that age where the child is undergoing full-time education or training or there are other special circumstances (s.5(3)(*b*)). Liability to make payment ceases on the payer's death. Special provision is however made by the 1978 Act to apply Part V of the 1980 Act where the child has attained the age of sixteen and is engaged in full-time remunerative work. Where this is the case the child will become the person liable for contributions towards his maintenance in accordance with section 45 of the Child Care Act 1980.

(ii) *Divorce Court orders*. When an order committing the child to the care of the local authority is made under section 43 of the Matrimonial Causes Act 1973, the court may order that the financial provision orders for children, available under the Act, be made in favour of the authority or to the child himself. This can include an order for periodical payments in accordance with the guidelines laid down in section 25 which direct the court to have regard to such matters as the financial needs of the child, any physical or mental disability of the child, and the manner in which he was being educated or trained. Such orders cease on the death of the person liable to make payment.

DURATION. Orders made under these provisions do not extend in the first instance beyond the child attaining the age of 17, unless the court specifies a later date, and should not extend beyond 18 in any case, unless the child is undergoing full-time education or training, or there are special circumstances when there is no limit.

(d) *Under wardship*

Where a child has been made a ward of court and committed into the care of the local authority, the court has power by virtue of section 6(2) of the Family Law Reform Act 1969 to order either or both parents to pay maintenance to the local authority. Maintenance may take the form of either weekly or periodical payments for the upkeep and education of the children as the court thinks reasonable having regard to the means of the person or persons on whom the requirement is imposed.

DURATION. The orders made under this Act extend in the first instance until the child ceases to be a minor (*i.e.* 18 years of age) unless they are earlier revoked, but can be extended only up to the age of 21 upon the application of the child or the local authority upon the same conditions as the earlier order was made.

B. Maintenance of children not technically "in care"

When a child is received into care under section 2 or is the subject of a care order or committal to care, that child may be placed in a local authority, controlled or assisted community home, a private children's home, a voluntary children's home, a hospital or a special school, but in some cases children may be placed in one of these institutions without any court orders or legislative procedure having been pursued, and the issue of maintenance is then a little more complex. The position of mentally handicapped children who may be placed in community homes without being received into care so that their parents are not required to make contributions is discussed later. (See below, Part II). The remaining problems concern children left by their parents in children's homes, or who have to remain in long-stay hospitals, or who have to attend special schools, because they are physically handicapped.

(a) *Children placed in voluntary homes*

Should parents for whatever reason place their child in a voluntary home with the organisation's consent, there is no legislation empowering the organisation to require contributions from the parent. Indeed, the definition in the 1980 Act of the voluntary home would appear to exclude even the possibility, since the home must be one "supported wholly or partly by voluntary contributions or endowments." Parents may choose to make contributions to the organisation to defray any part of the expenses incurred in looking after their children, and in that case, the home's status as a voluntary home would be unaffected.

In practice very few if any children are placed directly with voluntary organisations in their homes. Most placements in voluntary homes occur after referral through the social services departments, and even where parents directly approach the voluntary organisation with a request, it is customary for the organisation to refer them in the first place to the social services department for the area in which they live. Organisations like Barnardo's now seem themselves as providing alternative specialist or back-up facilities to local authorities, and thus nearly all of the children placed with them will have been received into care under section 2 or will have been committed into care, or less frequently be the subject of the 1969 Act care orders. The exceptions to this are mentally handicapped children placed by the local authority, who have come into their care under the Mental Health legislation.

Where accommodation run by a voluntary organisation is used by the local authority to provide a home for a child, arrangements are made between the local authority and the organisation concerned for the payment of expenses incurred in providing care and accommodation for the child.

A voluntary organisation may, however, be able to apply for child benefit in respect of a child who has nonetheless been placed directly with them. A voluntary organisation can be regarded as a person with whom the child is living for any week when he is living in premises managed by the organisation, or even where boarded out by it. (Child Benefit Regulations 1976). Ogus and Barendt (1978) comment that the eligibility of an organisation for benefit in this way seems to be unique in the social security system; there is no clear reason why it was decided to depart from the general rule that only natural persons are entitled. A voluntary organisation will not be so entitled however on the alternative basis that it is contributing to the cost of providing for the child (see below, p. 94). Under no circumstances is a local authority entitled to claim child benefit.

(b) *Physically handicapped children in special schools*

If it is impossible for a physically handicapped child to be educated in an ordinary school and he is assessed as having a special education need under section 1 of the Education Act 1981, and in consequence has to attend a special boarding school because of his disability, the obligation to pay the full cost of the boarding school falls on the local education authority (Education Act 1944, s.52(1)(*a*), as amended).

(c) *Other children in special boarding schools*

Similar provisions apply whereby pursuant to the Education Act 1981 a child is assessed as having a particular educational need, which can only be met by his attendance at a special school with boarding facilities (Education Act 1981, ss.1, 2).

(d) *Children in long-stay hospitals*

Where a child who for whatever reason has been received into hospital and subsequently remains there other than under local authority care provisions, there is no power in anyone to order that the parents should contribute directly towards his maintenance. This is basically because of the state-provided National Health Service, and parents in work or who have worked will have contributed to this service through deduction from their wages of the National Health insurance contribution.

(e) *Children in detention or in legal custody*

There is no power to order parents to make contributions towards the maintenance of any of their children in legal custody, whether they be held in detention centres, remand centres, prisons or even exceptionally where they are held in a community home pending final disposition.

II. *Social Security Benefits and Maintenance of Children in Residential Care*

A. Children in care of local authority

General

Where a child is received or committed into the care of the local authority under any of the provisions described above, the family's income may be substantially affected by adjustments which can in consequence be made to any of the benefits available through the state social security system.

Child benefit

Child benefit is payable to any person who in that week has the child living with him or is contributing to his maintenance at a weekly rate not lower than the rate of benefit (Child Benefit Act 1975, ss.1, 3(1)). The Act and the regulations issued thereunder provide that for the first eight weeks after a child has come into the care of the local authority, benefit will continue to be paid irrespective of the whereabouts of the child. After the first eight weeks entitlement depends upon whether the child comes home for visits and how long such visits last.

Benefit will continue to be paid in the usual way if a child "ordinarily lives with the person claiming benefit for at least one day each week." (Child Benefit (General) Regulations 1976, reg. 16(6)). So, if there are regular arrangements for the child to leave residential care for visits home each week that may be sufficient for entitlement to continue, provided the visit is for a period greater than one day. This is defined by the Adjudications Officer as a period of 24 hours from midnight to midnight. Effectively this means that a child must be at home for two consecutive nights each week in order for the parent to claim. This interpretation was however successfully challenged by a mother whose sons in care were at home from 1.00 p.m. on Saturday to 5.30 p.m. on Sunday each weekend, (*C.I.O. file 1.0.16 (MB./79*)) although Morgan (1981) reports another case in the same year where the Commissioner reached a different conclusion on very similar facts and disallowed a claim (*C.F., 35/1979*). According to DHSS instructions where a child normally goes home for weekends but is prevented from doing so occasionally, this should not affect the payment of benefit (*DHSS*, 1980).

A child who is allowed home from residential care for an occasional visit lasting longer than one week will entitle his parents to child benefit, and a fresh claim for benefit should be submitted by the parent. (reg. 16(6) and see *Lister*, 1981).

It is crucial to note that while it is up to parents to notify the child benefit authorities when a child comes home for visits and they are seeking to claim benefit for those periods, it is social workers who are responsible for notifying the child benefit centre five weeks after a child comes into care, and on discharge from care.

If, on the other hand, the parent is contributing to the child's maintenance at a rate equivalent to the benefit rate, child benefit is still payable. Since a large number of parents with children in residential care do not make contributions and no contribution orders have been made against them, this provision is likely to be applicable only to a small number of parents. If even a semblance of a system of agreed contributions or orders is to be maintained, it would seem sensible to suggest that where parents are receiving child benefit and their child goes into the care of the local authority, a contribution exactly equal to the amount of child benefit should be agreed between the parties, thus allowing parents to feel that they are at least contributing in some way to their child's upbringing.

Family Income Supplement

Family Income Supplement is, as its name implies, a supplement paid to families after submitting to a means test, where the bread-winner is in full-time work but their income is less than the level prescribed under the Family Income Supplements Act 1970. In order to qualify as a family there must be at least one child who is a member of the household *and* supported in whole *or in part* by the claimant. These conditions are strictly interpreted so that a child is not part of the household unless living under the same roof as the claimant who cannot be considered to be supporting the child unless the local authority actually requires the claimant to make a contribution towards the child's upkeep. According to Tunnard (1980) the strict interpretation of these conditions was successfully challenged in a local Supplementary Benefit Appeal Tribunal by a woman whose son, who was in residential care, normally came home for weekends and holidays. She was responsible for his upkeep while he was at home and for occasional clothing and other expenses whilst he was away. As a result of that case the former Chairman of the Supplementary Benefits Commission, David Donnison, commented that there would be some cases where a child should be regarded as part of the claimant's household for F.I.S. purposes, even though the child lives for much of the time in residential care (*Lister*, 1981). The onus is however on the claim-ant to show why the child should be treated as part of the house-hold and an example of how this can be established can be seen from the case of *England and England* v. *Secretary of State for Social Services* (1982). In that case the parents were both forced to go out to work to maintain their family and placed their children in voluntary care. The children were provided with residential accommodation and schooling during the week and returned home at weekends and in school holidays. The parents took care to keep their house as the children's home and retained the bedrooms for their use. In addition to the food, heating, lighting, furniture and bedding they provided toys, books and sporting equipment for the children and demonstrated to the children that they cared. They made efforts to pay the parental contributions required by the authority but were unable to make payment in full. The High

Court found that a claim for F.I.S. for the year in question should have been allowed.

Supplementary Benefit

According to the Supplementary Benefit (Amendment) Act 1976 and the Aggregation Regulations 1981, a claimant will only qualify for benefit on those days when the child is at home. Thus, if the child is allowed home on one day a week one-seventh of the weekly scale rate for a child of that age will be payable, and any balance of five hours or more counts as an additional twenty-four hours. When calculating the hours, time spent travelling to and from the residential home is counted. It is advisable for the claimant to notify the local social security office well in advance of those days when the child is to be at home; otherwise, there may well be endless delays in obtaining the extra benefit. Parents on supplementary benefit get no increase to their benefit in respect of those expenses which they may incur in visiting a child of theirs in care. However, section 26 of the Child Care Act 1980, gives local authorities the power to defray such expenses if it appears to them that the parents could not make such visits without undue hardship and the circumstances warrant payment.

Social Security benefits generally

If the parent is drawing unemployment, sickness or industrial injuries benefit, entitlement to the child's "dependant's increases" is conditional upon proving entitlement to child benefit in the same week. So, if they qualify for child benefit (see above, p. 94) the parents should also receive the relevant increases.

Mobility allowance

This benefit is payable to those over the age of five and under 65 suffering from physical disablement such that they are either unable to walk or virtually unable to walk. Under the regulations made pursuant to the introduction of mobility allowance; the allowance will in respect of a child between the ages of five and 15, who is in residential care, be paid to the person with whom the child is living who must give an undertaking to use it for the child's benefit. The benefit, somewhat unusually, therefore follows the child wherever he may be living (Mobility Allowance Regulations 1975). The parent may still qualify however where there is some contact between him and the child but this will be determined in accordance with the priority rules. (Mobility Allowance Regulations 1975).

Attendance allowance

This allowance is payable to a person who is so severely disabled, physically or mentally, that he requires either frequent attention throughout the day and prolonged or repeated attention during the night or continual supervision from another person in order to avoid substantial danger to himself or others. Following the first four weeks in care the parents are disqualified from claiming the allowance, unless they are contributing to the cost of providing for the child at a weekly rate of at least the amount of the attendance allowance and on top of any contribution required for entitlement to child benefit or increases to a contributory benefit. The local authority, or any other body with whom the child has his home, *e.g.* Barnardo's, is unable to qualify for the allowance in lieu of the parents. This was decided in a case argued by Barnardo's in 1975 before the Attendance Allowance Board (*R(A)* 3/75).

B. Children in special schools and long-stay hospitals who are not "in care"

While the automatic disqualification from benefits on the ground that the child is in care does not operate in the case of these children, the ordinary qualifying conditions for each of the benefits must be satisfied before the claimant is able to establish entitlement. Thus, for child benefit and any of the dependant increases for social security benefits, benefits will be unaffected where the parent is regularly contributing to the maintenance of the child at a rate equal to the amount of the benefit. In the case of a child in hospital, once the initial 12 weeks adjustment period is completed, benefits can still be claimed where the applicant is regularly incurring expenditure on the child, which may take the form of visits, purchasing of fruit, drinks, books and presents. Following the *England* decision (see above, p. 96) it is suggested that family income supplement could still be claimed where the child is a long-stay patient in a hospital, but comes home for weekends and the parents are incurring regular expenditure in maintaining contact with the child.

The rules for supplementary benefit are similar to those applicable for child benefit thus if the claimant is eligible for a child benefit in respect of a child away at a special school (on the basis of contributions or residence for part of the week, see above, pp. 94–95), the child can be included in the claimant's assessment. Where the child is in hospital for a period in excess of twelve weeks, the dependant's increase is reduced to a fixed amount of approximately one-fifth of the normal rate, although additions can be given to the claimant for fares to visit the child (*DHSS*, 1981).

As already indicated, mobility allowance follows the child and thus can still be paid for a child in a long-stay hospital provided he will benefit from an enhancement of the facilities for locomotion, provided by payment of the allowance (Social Security Act 1975, s.37A(2)(*d*)). Attendance allowance is not payable to an institution or organisation, and where the child is in hospital the rules against overlapping of benefits would prevent payment to parents in such circumstances as the National Health Service has responsibility for the care of the child.

C. Children undergoing imprisonment or detention in legal custody

Entitlement to child benefit and thus to dependant's increases to social security benefits are in the case of children undergoing imprisonment or detention in legal custody, governed by the provision of Schedule 1 of the Child Benefit Act 1975. As is the case with children made the subjects of care orders, child benefit continues to be payable for the first eight weeks. Disqualification from entitlement to child benefit and to the other dependant's increases will therefore arise once the child has been in a detention centre or other form of legal custody for periods in excess of eight weeks (Child Benefit Regulations 1976, reg. 16(6)). Where the parents are in receipt of supplementary benefit the DHSS should be informed and no increase will be payable in respect of the child for the period of detention or custody since the child will have no supplementary benefit requirements (*DHSS*, 1980). However, additions to benefit can be made to enable parents to visit children in legal custody and in detention centres (*DHSS*, 1980).

5. Day-Care Establishments for Children

Introduction

For a large number of parents permanent residential substitute care is not the solution to the problem of what to do with their children during the day. In respect of many children under five, difficulty arises because their mothers either want or need to go out to work, but for a few the problems may arise because the child is handicapped in some way, or the parent is in poor health, and the parent needs a break or some assistance during the day. The solution for the former group is some form of day nursery or child minding provision and for the latter it may take the form of day-nursery or some other specialised form of day care provision such as a nursery school for handicapped children. Some parents simply want their children to have pre-school education or play experience and for these groups nursery classes and schools and also play-groups provide or would provide what is required.

Day-nurseries and nursery classes and school places may be provided by local authorities but a number are provided by private institutions. These are subject to a certain degree of control. Child minding facilities are provided entirely by individuals some of whom are registered with the local authority, though the vast majority probably are not (*Central Policy Review Staff*, 1978). Registration ensures a limited degree of control over child minders actually on the register. There has also been a considerable growth in the number of play-groups which are subject to the same registration requirement, unless eligible for special exemption. In the case of children with special needs, the Education Acts 1944–1981 provide that local education authorities ought to provide special education for any such child at any age, although it is not compulsory for parents to take it up until the child is five years old. Since the policy is to give priority to cases of particular need when allocating day nursery places, parents of a handicapped child under two, who find it difficult to manage all day every day, should not have too much trouble in establishing their need for a place or the local education authority may itself direct that a child be placed in such a day nursery. (Education Act 1981, s.3).

In this section the law relating to the provision, regulation and cost of all forms of day care for children is examined. The legal implication for all those involved is also discussed.

I. *Nursery Schools and Nursery Classes*

Provision

Since educational provision generally is outside the scope of this work, the position of nursery schools and classes will only be briefly discussed. Nursery education is defined in the Education Act 1944 as education for children over two and under five, which may be provided in nursery schools, or in the nursery classes of primary schools. (s.9(4)). In terms of the number of places available nursery education in this country is woefully inadequate. (*Statistics of Education,* 1979). The war years saw a certain expansion as mothers were encouraged to work and the 1944 Act built on this by providing that, in fulfilling their duty to provide sufficient schools in their area, a local education authority should in particular have regard to the need for securing provision for the under-fives in nursery schools or, where this was inexpedient, in nursery classes (s.8(2)). In other words, the provision of nursery education was not compulsory and little progress was made. The Plowden Report (1967) recommended the expansion of nursery education particularly in those areas designated "educational priority areas" and this was followed by the Government's Urban Aid Programme aimed at areas of special social need which in the first five years allocated resources for nursery education. After a period in which responsibility for providing nursery education was shifted to the local education authorities, as a result of the Education White

Paper, resources were again made available from the Urban Aid Programme in 1977. Despite all this support the economic climate has not encouraged expansion and the further cutbacks in the nursery education programme mean that demand for nursery school places will continue to exceed supply. The possibility for any real growth in the provision of nursery education received a further setback in 1980 with the repeal of section 8(2) of the Education Act 1944 and its replacement with the much weaker section 24 of the Education Act 1980. Thus, instead of the local education authority being required to have regard to the need for nursery provision in discharging its duty to provide sufficient schools, the emasculated provisions emphasise that the local education authority shall not be under any duty to provide education for children under five (s.24(2)) and further they simply have the *power* to establish nursery schools (s.24(1)).

Local authority nursery education provision falls into two categories, nursery classes and nursery schools. Nursery classes are generally for children over three but not yet five and are usually attached to a school, the majority of whose pupils are over five. Where a nursery class is part of such a school, it has two sessions in the morning and the afternoon, starting at the same time as the rest of the school but over half the children in such classes will attend for one session only. This is in line with the policy of successive governments to encourage part-time rather than full-time education for children below the age of five on the grounds that it is not only cheaper but actually preferable. (*Stone and Taylor*, 1976).

Nursery schools on the other hand are used chiefly for the education of two to five year olds and so, for example, they can be used to discharge the local education authority's responsibility in respect of the education of children with special needs. The government has had the power since 1918 to make grants in respect of local authority nursery schools. As well as the nursery schools and classes provided by the state, there are a large number of independent nursery schools which fill some of the gap left by the inadequacy of state provision, though only for those who can afford it.

Regulation

The Schools Regulations 1959, as amended, provide that

children not be admitted to a state nursery class under the age of three nor allowed to stay after the end of the term in which they have their fifth birthday unless exceptional circumstances require it. The same provision operates in relation to state nursery schools except that the admission range is two and five (reg.7). These schools and classes are provided, inspected and controlled by local education authorities, and thus being subject to the Schools Regulations are exempt from registration under the Nurseries and Child Minders Regulation Act 1948 (s.8(3)). Where the nursery school is run by a private individual or body, it may be required to be registered with the Department of Education and Science and will be classified as a school, in which case it will be subject to inspection by the local education authority. Alternatively, it may be classified as a playgroup and in that case will be registered with and inspected by the local social services department, in accordance with the provisions of the Nurseries and Child Minders Regulation Act 1948 (hereafter the 1948 Act). Classification will depend on the extent to which education as such is provided over and above simply placing the child in an environment where there is opportunity to play with other children.

Payment

Where the nursery school or nursery class place is provided by the local education authority, there is no charge for parents of children. In the case of independent nursery schools, charges are made and vary enormously. There is no limit on the amount which can be charged.

II. *Day Nurseries, Play Groups and Child Minders*

Provision

Day nurseries generally take babies from the age of six months up to the age at which they start school. Whether they are provided by the social services authorities or by private bodies they are usually open for those hours in which parents would be expected to be at work, and they do not shut during school holidays. Where the day nurseries are run by or under the auspices of the social services department they tend to give priority to cases of particular need, *e.g.* single parent families and families where parents or children are handicapped in some way. Occasionally, children will be placed in a local authority day nursery following the directions of a juvenile court, where a parent has agreed to supervision pursuant to the institution of care proceedings. The purpose of local authority day nurseries is thus to provide a social service for families rather than to educate children, though the staff will normally be familiar with all aspects of child care. By section 26 of the Education Act 1980, local education authorities may now make available to a day nursery the services of any teacher who is employed by them in a nursery class or school, and who agrees to provide his services to the day nursery. A number of day nurseries are also provided by private individuals or bodies. Terry (1979) states that in 1944 when day nurseries were a national necessity, to enable women to work in essential industries, there were 72,000 local authority day nursery places. However, this figure had fallen to 30,500 full-time and 4,700 part-time places by 1976. The number of places available in registered private nurseries in the same year was 26,000.

In addition to the maintained and independent sectors the voluntary sector provides a much needed service in the form of play groups. Play groups rely heavily on parental involvement though the leader would be expected to have a playleader's qualification. As Stone and Taylor point out (1976) play groups not only offer children under five good play materials, space, stimulation and companionship, they may also offer support, companionship and education to the mothers who help in running them. Some play groups are independent but the vast majority receive grants from the local education authority or from the social services department. Most play groups will only accept children for one session a day, either the morning of afternoon for a couple of hours, and some further restrict attendance to two or three days a week.

While the number of places in state day nurseries and nursery schools continues to be so low, the costs in equivalent private institutions so high, and the period of the day covered by play groups so inadequate, for most parents the only day care option is to place their child with a child minder. Statistics would seem to indicate that this is the most widely used substitute day care arrangement made by parents who have to be at work all day. Research studies have shown that mothers viewed child minding as the least satisfactory form of day care, and would have preferred to place their child in a local authority day nursery, (*Bone*, 1976) and that mothers might be unhappy about the minder they used but reluctant to move their children because of lack of alternative facilities or any guarantee that a different child minder would be any better (*Mayall and Petrie*, 1977).

A child minder is a person who for reward (in cash or in kind) receives children under five into her home to be looked after for the day, or for part or parts of the day, if it amounts to more than two hours, or for any longer period not exceeding six days. Any child minder should be registered with the local authority under the Nurseries and Child Minders Regulation Act 1948 but the registration requirement is notoriously difficult to enforce. The controls laid down by the 1948 Act really only attempt the imposition of minimal standards of control, and registration may also be useful in advertising minders and indicating to parents the range of options available. Some child minders operate entirely on their own while others employ assistance. Indeed, where the minder has the care of more than three children, including any of her own below school age, then official guidance suggests that additional help *should* be employed. (*Ministry of Health*, 1968).

Despite the registration requirement, there is, as indicated, evidence to suggest that illegal minding is quite prevalent (*Jackson and Jackson*, 1979), and, as Hoggett (1981) points out, evidence for prosecution for failure to register is "hard to obtain, the victims are too young to complain, their hard-pressed parents do not want to, and social workers cannot make regular house to house checks." Terry (1979) has suggested that much more positive encouragement should be given to child minders to seek registration. Thus, she argues, a successful applicant could be offered training courses, advice and even financial assistance for the provision of equipment. An application for registration could then be seen as a step towards obtaining many possible advantages instead of as inviting the risk of losing a livelihood and the danger of prosecution. These additional incentives would at least entail a recognition of the very real social service which the child minders provide (*Jackson and Jackson*, 1979) and would widen the scope of the protection afforded by the 1948 Act.

Regulation

Day nurseries, play groups and child minders are controlled alike by the registration and inspection provisions of the 1948 Act, as amended by section 60 of the Health Services and Public Health Act 1968 and the Local Government Act 1972. Any premises which are provided or assisted by local social services or are controlled in other ways are however exempt from the operation of the 1948 Act (s.8(3)).

The 1948 Act differentiates between the need to register premises and the need to register persons. Every local social services authority must keep registers of premises (excluding private dwellings) where children are received to be looked after for the day or part of the day; in addition, a register must be kept of people in the area who, for reward, receive children into their homes to be looked after on a daily basis (s.1). The registers must be open to inspection at all reasonable times (s.1).

Anyone wishing to receive children into a nursery or child minding position may apply to the social services authority for registration, which is subject to:

(a) the person employed or proposed to be employed to look after the children being a fit person to do so;

(b) the premises used or proposed to be used being fit to be used, in terms of their condition, equipment, situation, construction or size.

An application for registration of any premises must contain a statement with respect to each person employed or proposed to be employed in looking after children at the premises, and each person who is 16 years or older who is normally resident at the premises. The application for registration of a person must contain a similar clause.

Registration requirements

The social services department may restrict the number of children to be received into the premises registered with them, or to be looked after by persons registered with them (s.2(1)). Registration may also include the requirement that precautions be taken against the exposing of children to infectious diseases. In registering premises, the authority may impose conditions as to the qualifications of the person in charge and other staff (s.2(4)(*a*)), the level of staffing (s.2(4)(*b*)), repairs and alterations to premises (s.2(4)(*c*)), safety and maintenance of the premises and equipment (s.2(4)(*d*)), arrangements for feeding children (s.2(4)(*e*)), medical supervision of children (s.2(4)(*f*)) and the records to be kept in relation to the children (s.2(4)(*g*)).

Provided the authority is satisfied, a certificate registering a person or premises for receiving children will be issued. This may be revoked or varied subsequently by the authority. Failure to register or to abide by the conditions of registration is a criminal offence, and a person found guilty can be fined or imprisoned (s.4). Where a person who is registered to receive children moves house, the registration lapses automatically until notice is given to the local social services department (s.4(3)).

Appeals

Where the local social services authority intends to refuse, cancel or impose requirements on registration, they must give 14 days notice to the occupier of the premises, or to the person seeking registration or already registered (s.6). The grounds will be stated and the applicant, occupier or person must have the opportunity to give reasons why the refusal, cancellation or imposing of conditions should not happen. If he or she is dissatisfied with the result, he may appeal to a court of summary jurisdiction, or in Scotland to the Sheriff (s.6(4)). In the case of the proposed cancellation of an existing registration, this is not to be executed whilst an appeal is pending (s.6(4)).

Inspection

Anyone authorised by the local social services department to do so, may enter registered premises in that area at any reasonable time (s.7(1)). The person may inspect the premises and the children received within them and the arrangements made for their welfare and any records kept (s.7(1)). The person has similar powers in respect of the home of any person registered by the local authority (s.7(1)). Where the authorised person has reason to believe that children are being received into a person's home or other premises which are not registered, the inspector may apply to a magistrate (or Sheriff in Scotland) for a warrant authorising entry to the house or premises to carry out an inspection (s.7(2)).

Payment for Substitute Day Care

Nursery schools and nursery classes

When these are provided by the local education authority pursuant to their power under the Education Acts there is no charge. Parents placing their children in independent nursery schools must clearly expect to pay the charges stipulated, though occasionally a child may be placed by the local education authority in an independent nursery school, in which case the parent does not have to pay.

Day nurseries

Where the day nursery places are provided by a local social services authority under the powers granted by the National Health Service Act 1977, they are also able to make reasonable charges for such places according to the parents' means (Sched. 8, para. 1). Thus, some limit is set to the fees payable. If the day nursery is private, there is no restriction on the charges made to parents.

Play groups

Whether play groups are run by voluntary groups or are assisted or controlled by the education authority or social services departments, they normally make a small charge to cover running and administrative costs.

Child minders

Generally, child minders offer their services for cash but some are prepared to accept payment in kind. Their charges are directly related to what the market in the particular vicinity will bear, and since child minders have few, if any, capital costs, they probably provide the cheapest full-time substitute day care. It has been proposed (*Ministry of Health*, 1968) that a number of child minders could be paid by local authorities where they are willing to take on children from the local authority who fall within certain priority categories eligible for day care support, for example, single parents. In addition, the Health Services and Public Health Act 1968 empowers local authorities to pay child minders directly and to recover charges from the child's parents according to their means.

III. *Day-Care Provision for Juvenile Offenders*

There are basically two forms of day care provision for juvenile offenders, *i.e.* those children under the age of 17 who have been found guilty of a criminal offence, and these are intermediate treatment centres and attendance centres. Intermediate treatment centres may also be used under the terms of a supervision order, made when a child fulfils the conditions laid down in section 1(1)(*a*)–(*e*) of the Children and Young Persons Act 1969 and the court is of the opinion that such an order is the best means of dealing with the child. They can further be used under the terms of section 1 of the Child Care Act 1980 where such action is deemed necessary in order to diminish the need to receive the children into care. Intermediate treatment represents an attempt to shift the emphasis away from residential care and a commitment to the therapeutic ideal. Attendance centres are more in line with the punitive ideal widely supported by magistrates.

(a) Intermediate treatment centres

Provision

Since the passage of the Criminal Justice Act 1982, the power to direct that a child subject to a supervision order made in criminal proceedings should attend an intermediate treatment centre is one exercisable either by the supervisor though delegated to him by the court (C.Y.P.A. 1969, s.12(2)–(3), as amended by C.J.A. 1982, s.20), sometimes referred to as discretionary intermediate treatment, or by the court itself (C.Y.P.A. 1969, s.12(3A)–(3C), as amended by C.J.A. 1982, s.20), sometimes called the stipulated intermediate treatment requirement. Where intermediate treatment is being provided by virtue of the local authority's powers under section 1 of the Child Care Act 1980 it is not subject to any directions given by the court. The type of daytime facilities for intermediate treatment which may be provided at day centres (usually school or other local authority premises are set out in the early Department of Health and Social Security's guide to intermediate treatment (*DHSS*, 1972) and as a result of the changes made consequent upon the Criminal Justice Act 1982 in a Home Office Circular issued in 1983 (Home Office Circular No. 42/1983 paras. 53–55). All the facilities listed in a scheme for use pursuant to directions given under section 12 of the Children and Young Persons Act 1969 must be approved by, or of a type approved by the Secretary of State, and these are listed in the Appendix to the Circular. If a local authority wishes to include in a scheme facilities that are different from those specified in the list they are invited to write to Children's Division A, Alexander Fleming House, Elephant and Castle, London, S.E.1, with a brief description of the activities requesting the Secretary of State's approval. The sort of facilities listed are those which provide for one or more activities of a recreational, educational or cultural nature of social value, including but not limited to the following: physical education, competitive sports or games, adventure training, camping, cycling, walking, climbing, amateur dramatics, arts, crafts, remedial education, evening classes, group counselling, debating, community or social service projects and work experience. As with residential intermediate treatment, the facility should be provided by a responsible person or body specified in the scheme and at all times when making use of the facility in accordance with directions given either by the supervisor or the court under sections 12(2)–(3A–3C) of the 1969 Act, the supervised person will be under the charge and control of the supervisor or some other responsible person.

Regulation

The new arrangements made under the Criminal Justice Act 1982 are clearly intended to strengthen the supervision order by empowering the courts to specify participation in a particular programme of intermediate treatment activities. Under the previous arrangements when the form which treatment took was solely at the discretion of the supervisor, official guidance emphasised the need to involve the child and his family when deciding a suitable programme of activities (*DHSS*, 1977). This guidance still applies to what has been called discretionary intermediate treatment. Before the court stipulates a particular programme of intermediate treatment however, it is now required by the statute to:

(a) consult the prospective supervisor as to the offender's circumstances and as to the feasibility of securing compliance with the requirements.

(b) to consider that having regard to the circumstances of the case the requirements are necessary for securing the good conduct of the supervised person or for preventing a repetition by him of the same offence or the commission of other offences;

and finally to

(c) secure the consent of the supervised person, or where he is under 14, of his parent or guardian, to the inclusion of the intermediate treatment requirements.

Once the course of intermediate treatment has begun, frequent reviews are desirable. A review shortly after the start provides an opportunity to establish the suitability of the programme selected and in the case of discretionary treatment allows for the supervisor to make modifications. Thereafter, the DHSS suggests that regular reviews are necessary to assess progress, confirm the continuing suitability of the programme and to monitor the general effectiveness of particular activities. Where the child undergoing intermediate treatment is on a supervision order, the supervisor is required to keep in touch with those running the facilities and to ask for regular reports, (*DHSS*, 1977). If the child fails to fulfil his obligations there is no real sanction unless the original supervision order was made in criminal proceedings. In those circumstances were the child then to fail to comply with the order for intermediate treatment, the sanctions for such breach include a fine of up to £50 or an attendance centre order (Criminal Law Act 1977, s.37). The supervision order thus increasingly begins to look like the probation order which it replaced. A potentially more drastic step open to the supervisor, where the order was made in criminal proceedings, would be to seek the substitution of a care order (C.Y.P.A. 1969, s.15) and see above p. 52).

Because of the variegated nature of intermediate treatment provision, there can be no rules or regulations governing the conduct of centres at which activities may be run. More generalised guidance as to the scope and organisation facilities issues from time to time in circulars. One of these (*DHSS*, 1977) emphasised that "a successful intermediate treatment programme should considerably reduce the need for residential care providing in many cases a more suitable form of treatment at potentially less cost," and pointed out that a modest switch of resources from residential treatment to intermediate treatment would represent a very substantial increase in resources for intermediate treatment. Leeding (1980) states that although there has been increasing investment in intermediate treatment, it is not so far known to what extent it has been successful in its objectives. Despite lack of evidence as to the success of intermediate treatment, the changes just described represent an attempt to encourage the courts to make greater use of intermediate treatment. The powers given to the courts in the amended section 12(3)(A–C) of the Children and Young Persons Act 1969 by the Criminal Justice Act 1982 were effected in order to persuade courts to choose intermediate treatment as a realistic, alternative sentencing option. The White Paper (1980 para. 50) which preceded the Bill suggested that if the courts knew what the programme was to be, they would have more confidence in the order. McEwan (1983), however, justifiably suggests that the Government would have been well advised to look more closely at the reason behind the reluctance of social workers to recommend the supervision order, since there is considerable evidence that their lack of faith is responsible, at least in part, for the decline in the use made by the courts of such orders. (*Giller and Morris*, 1981; *Parker, Casburn and Turnbull*, 1981). A more recent circular emphasises the factors which local authorities should bear in mind when developing facilities in response to the new arrangements. (*DHSS*, 1983). Thus, the circular states that "local authorities will clearly wish to bear in mind that courts may not consider offenders participation in intermediate treatment programmes as an effective alternative to custody, unless suitable programmes are available and they have confidence in them. They will clearly wish to make use of the opportunity provided by the new requirement for them to draw up schemes of intermediate treatment facilities in consultation with the probation service, to give high priority to the development of suitable intermediate treatment facilities for inclusion in these schemes. Cooperation with all concerned—statutory or voluntary agencies—and close liaison with courts is likely to result in the provision of facilities which command local confidence" (*DHSS*, 1983 para. 19).

Payment

In order to finance the necessary increased provision of new facilities, the Government announced early in 1983 that 15 million pounds would be made available for extending intermediate treatment. The increased funding is available to all local authorities who develop facilities under the revised scheme (see above, p. 82) and they generally bear responsibility for meeting the costs of intermediate treatment. The only expenditure therefore required to be met by parents is the possible cost of fares to and from the centre.

(b) Attendance centres

Provision

Attendance centres are designed to deal with young offenders whose future conduct may be expected to be influenced by the deprivation of leisure time involved and by the endeavour of staff to encourage them to make constructive use of leisure time and to guide them towards worthwhile recreational activities, which they can continue on leaving the centre (*Sentence of the Court*, 1978).

Unlike intermediate treatment establishments, attendance centres are part of the penal system and thus come under the control of the Home Office and not of local authorities or the DHSS. As a form of treatment for young offenders they were introduced by the Criminal Justice Act 1948. This Act authorised the Home Secretary to provide attendance centres for offenders of not less than 12 but under 21 years and to issue rules for their management and regulation. The lower age limit was reduced to ten by the Criminal Justice Act 1961.

Attendance centre orders can be made by the courts in respect of any offence punishable in the case of an adult by imprisonment (C.J.A. 1982, s.17(1)) and under the new provisions may be imposed even where the offender has previously been sentenced to custody, including borstal training, youth custody or detention centre, where it appears to the court that there are special circumstances relating either to the offence or to the offender which may justify the making of an order (C.J.A. 1982, s.17(3)). Both the magistrates' courts and the Crown Court now have the power to make an attendance centre order (C.J.A. 1982, s.16(2)) whereas previously the Crown Court's powers were more restricted. These courts can also make attendance centre orders for non-payment of a fine or for a breach of a requirement included in a supervision order made in criminal proceedings (C.J.A. 1982, s.17(1)(*a*) and see above, p. 83).

The recent legislation provides that the aggregate number of hours of attendance ordered should not generally exceed 12 hours unless the court is of the opinion that 12 hours would be inadequate, in which case if the offender is aged between 14 and 17 it cannot exceed 24 hours, or if over 17, 36 hours (C.J.A. 1982, s.17(5)). Where the offender is under 14 then the aggregate should be not less than 12 hours, unless the court is of the opinion that such would be excessive, having regard to his age and circumstances. (C.J.A. 1982, s.17(4)). The courts are now further given the power to make an attendance centre order before a previous order has expired without regard to the number of hours in the previous order (C.J.A. 1982, s.17(6)). In addition the power to discharge and vary an attendance centre order is extended to the magistrates' court which made the order (s.18(3)(*b*)) and breach of an attendance centre order is now punishable by the court which made the order as well as the court in whose area the attendance centre is (C.J.A. 1982, s.19(2)). The order is designed to interfere with the child's leisure time and not with school or working hours. Accordingly, attendance is normally required on Saturdays for up to a maximum of three hours. No order should be made unless the court is satisfied that the attendance centre is reasonably accessible to the person concerned having regard to his age, the means of access available to him and any other circumstances.

There are currently some 80 junior attendance centres (for those under 17) and two senior attendance centres (for those over 17 but under 21) for boys, and two junior centres for girls (aged 14 to 17) (*Home Office*, 1977). Since the attendance centre order has proved so popular ever since their introduction (*McClintock*, 1961; *Dunlop*, 1980) plans have been made for several more, including another centre for girls to be situated in Greater London (*Home Office*, 1979).

The responsibility for providing attendance centres rests with the Home Office, usually by arrangement with the police in each area though in some places for example Hull and Plymouth, the Director of Social Services deals with the supervision of centres (*Home Office*, 1977). Centres are run by people such as school teachers, serving or retired policemen, and very often the premises on which they are held are schools with a gym and showers, boys clubs, or police premises such as police training schools.

Regulation

Attendance centres are currently subject to the Attendance Centre Rules 1958 and the Amendment Rules 1983 which provide for such matters as the keeping of registers and the discipline to be observed in the centre. The Criminal Justice Act 1982 provided that the Secretary of State could make further rules for the regulation and management of attendance centres. Discipline is under the control of the officer in charge and the staff (r. 7) and every person attending the centre must conduct himself in an orderly manner and obey any order given by that officer or any member of staff (r. 8). Failure to attend the centre, or breach of any of the rules can result in the offender being brought back to court, and the court may deal with him in any way in which he could have been dealt with in the original proceedings (C.J.A. 1982, s.19(8)).

The Home Office regards the purpose of the attendance centre order as being: (i) to vindicate the law by imposing loss of leisure; (ii) to bring the offender for a period under the influence of representatives of the authority of the state; (iii) to teach him something of the constructive use of leisure (*Home Office*, 1979). Research would tend to suggest that, while the first two aims are generally appreciated by the boys, both boys and staff were not convinced that the final aim was realised (*Dunlop, 1980*). Several officers in charge have expressed regrets that they are unable to include in the programme activities of greater interest and value to the boys, giving as examples: motor mechanics and do-it-yourself skills or tasks which would be useful to the community. The chief conclusions of Dunlop's study, however, were that junior attendance centres appeared to be satisfactorily achieving the objectives set by the courts, that they are used for a wide variety of offender, and that there are no contra-indications to their continued use for any particular type of boy. There is as yet no evidence as to their effectiveness in dealing with girls, since the two centres in Manchester and Middlesbrough only opened in 1979 (*Home Office*, 1979).

IV. *Legal Implications of Day-Care Provision*

Care and control of children

Where a child is placed by a parent, by an order of the court, or any other person for a day or any part of a day, the person into whose care the child is delivered will have certain responsibilities in respect of that child.

(a) *Care*

The Children and Young Persons Act 1933 provides that where any person who is legally liable to maintain a child fails to provide adequate food, clothing, medical aid or lodging for the child, he will be deemed to be guilty of a criminal offence (s.1). This provision covers local authority personnel in whose care a child has been placed and any independent person who undertakes in return for money to provide such services for the child during the day. Where an independent institution such as a day nursery is in breach of its contractual obligations to the parent, the parent could attempt to sue for breach of contract, and, where the child has suffered some injury, for damages in negligence. Were any cause for concern to arise at any establishment which requires to be registered with the local authority under the 1948 Act, this could be reported and registration can be cancelled (see above, pp. 18 and 20).

If it is thought that a child is not being adequately cared for at any establishment run by the local education authority, or the social services department, this too should be reported in the first instance to the department concerned, and then to the D.E.S. or DHSS, both of whom have their own inspectorate. Reports may also be made to the local police in serious cases, and further action such as an action in negligence or for breach of statutory duty may be considered.

Difficulties can also arise where a child in the care of a nursery school, day nursery, child minder or officer in charge of an intermediate treatment centre or attendance centre, has an accident. The person or body *in loco parentis* has a duty to take reasonable care of a child in their care (C.Y.P.A. 1933, s.1). Where the person actually looking after the child is an employee of someone else, for example the local education authority or independent nursery body, it is a basic principle of English law that the master is responsible for the negligence of his servant if the servant is acting in the course of his employment. Thus in *Carmarthenshire County Council* v. *Lewis* (1955), the council was held liable where a boy of four escaped when he was left on his own while attending a nursery school run by the council. He strayed out of the school and into the road, where a lorry driver swerving to avoid him was killed. The council was held liable to pay compensation under the Fatal Accidents Acts to the lorry driver's family, but the principle would have been the same had it been the child who had been killed or injured. The council, through its servant or agent, had been negligent and the council had to pay. Local education authorities and social services departments are usually protected against the cost of such claims by insurance policies, and independent persons running day care establishments should make certain that they are insured against these and other risks.

The general health and safety conditions for all persons employed on premises or liable to be affected are now governed by the provisions of the Health and Safety at Work Act 1974. In addition any premises provided by the local education authority must comply with the Schools Regulations 1959 in respect of danger from fire or other causes. The 1948 Act imposes similarly strict safety requirements for independently run premises. Failure to meet any of the requirements may lead to closure because the building does not possess adequate fire protection (Fire Precautions Act 1971) or cancellation of registration under the 1948 Act.

(b) *Control*

The Children and Young Persons Act 1933 gives any person having the lawful control or charge of a child or young person the right to administer punishment to the child (s.1(7)). Such punishment must however be reasonable and moderate, otherwise the person may render himself liable to prosecution for a criminal offence under the same act (s.1(2)).

Where a child temporarily in someone else's care commits a criminal offence the parent or guardian may still be held responsible for the child's acts in that if a court imposes a fine or costs or makes a compensation order in respect of the commission of such an offence by a child under 17, it can order that these be paid by the child's parent or guardian, though they must be given an opportunity to come to court and be heard on the matter (C.Y.P.A. 1933, s.55 and C.Y.P.A. 1969, s.3(6), as amended by C.J.A. 1982, ss.26–27). Under the amended provisions the court need not make any of these orders against a parent or guardian where it is satisfied that the parent or guardian cannot be found, or that in the circumstances of the case it would be unreasonable to make an order (C.Y.P.A. 1933, s.55(1) and C.Y.P.A. 1969, s.3(6)(*b*), as amended). In addition should the child commit a criminal offence whilst taking part in an intermediate treatment course, or when subject to an attendance centre order then he may find himself back before the court and liable to the imposition of a much heavier penalty. (see above, pp. 52 and 83).

Parents are not generally liable for their child's torts and thus someone *in loco parentis* would also not be liable, unless through the parents' or his substitute's negligence, the child has been given the opportunity of injuring or causing injury to another, the child's actions were reasonably foreseeable and a prudent parent would have taken precautions to forestall such a possibility (*Newton* v. *Edgerley*, 1959). Where the parent or his delegate had taken all reasonable steps then no liability arises (*Donaldson* v. *McNiven*, 1952). Should the parent or parent substitute however be found to have been negligent, he, or where relevant his employer, will be held liable in damages (*Carmarthenshire County Council* v. *Lewis*, 1955, see above, p. 62).

Difficulties may arise in this area for statutory bodies such as local authorities, who are supposed to be exercising control over a child pursuant to their statutory powers. Thus, if a child, either as part of an attendance centre order or as a participant in an intermediate treatment scheme, is directed towards activities which provide him with an opportunity to give vent to some known and potentially damaging proclivity, the statutory body may find itself responsible for the payment of damages in any negligence action which could result. Such a liability should, it has been argued, only arise where the decision made in exercise of the statutory powers was manifestly unreasonable or made in bad faith (*Home Office* v. *Dorset Yacht Co. Ltd.*, 1970), though just what can amount to such manifest unreasonableness is difficult to assess (see p. 62 and *McEwan*, 1980 and 1982).

Comment

A wide range of day care provision for children exists both within the public and private sectors, all of it subject to legal controls, more rigorously applied in some areas of provision than in others. At one end of the scale subject to the most tightly administered controls are the institutions provided by statutory bodies such as the local education authority or the Home Office, with independent day nurseries, registered child minders and voluntary play groups somewhere in the middle, and unregistered child minders at the other end of the scale escaping the controls, yet still providing day care for thousands of children. At a time of shrinking resources some might find it difficult perhaps to urge that more attention should be given to the problem of ensuring that all children in day-care are adequately protected from the risks of abuse or neglect. It should also not be assumed that simply because children are placed in an institutional setting, even one run by social services or the local education authority, that they are automatically safe. Greater control must be exercised over day-care provision especially at a time when an increasing number of mothers with children under school age are going out to work (*Social Trends*, 1981). In particular, the ever-increasing numbers of unregistered child minders should be positively encouraged to come in from the cold, more especially because successive governments seem to have been determined that state day-care provision should not be freely and extensively available. Even a small grant for expenditure on training, equipping and supervising child minders could result in a considerable return on the investment, an investment after all in the children of the society of today, the adults of its tomorrow.

Part II
The Mentally Disordered

6. Admission to Mental Hospitals

The law governing admission to mental hospitals is now governed by the Mental Health Act 1983 which has replaced the Mental Health Act 1959, amended by the Mental Health (Amendment) Act 1982, the provisions of which came into operation on September 30, 1983 (M.H.(A)A. 1982, s.69). The process of reform of the 1959 Act began in 1975 with the publication of the MIND report (*A Human Condition*) and of the Butler report on *Mentally Abnormal Offenders* (Cmnd. 6244). There was a Consultative Document published in 1976 by the Department of Health and Social Security (*A Review of the Mental Health Act 1959*) and a White Paper in 1978 (*Review of the Mental Health Act 1959*, Cmnd. 7320 (1978)). A further explanatory White Paper accompanied the Bill, when this was published in November 1981 (*Reform of Mental Health Legislation*, Cmnd. 8405). (On the historical background generally see *Jones*, 1972; *Gostin*, 1983; *Bean*, 1980). The 1983 Act consolidates the 1959 and 1982 Acts. References are only made to the earlier Acts where this is necessary for a complete understanding of the 1983 Act, or where they have not been replaced.

I. *Definitions*

The 1959 Act defined mental disorder as "mental illness, arrested or incomplete development of mind, psychopathic disorder, and any other disorder or disability of mind" (s.4(1)). This broad definition was not changed by the 1982 Act, except in so far as section

2(2) provided a limit to what constitutes mental disorder. Section 4(5) of the 1959 Act provided that a person is not to be treated as suffering from mental disorder by reason only of promiscuity or other immoral conduct. To this is now added "sexual deviancy or dependence on alcohol or drugs." (M.H.A. 1983, s.1(3)).

The 1959 Act, as amended by the 1982 Act (see now M.H.A. 1983, s.1), lists four specific categories of mental disorder which it is useful further to subdivide because different legal consequences may follow.

First, there is *mental illness*. This is nowhere defined by statute. The 1978 White Paper justified the absence of a definition in terms of the "difficulties of producing a definition that would stand the test of time" (*DHSS*, 1978). The problem with over-generalised concepts is that they can become "catch-all" categories. Thus, the fact that alcohol and drug dependency and sexual deviancy are no longer regarded as mental disorders may not prevent an "over-zealous treatment official" from finding "some associated condition, say reactive depression, or anxiety which justifies detention" (*Bean*, 1979, p. 101) (see also *Walker and McCabe*, 1973). The Percy Commission (*Law Relating to Mental Illness and Mental Deficiency*, 1957, Cmnd. 169) assumed that mental illness would be understood as "being of unsound mind" as "lunacy" had under previous legislation. The Butler report (1975) defines mental illness as a "disorder which has not always existed in the patient but has developed as a condition overlying the sufferer's usual personality." This is not of much assistance. The Court of Appeal has also tried to define mental illness. In *W*. v. *L*. (1974), which concerned a young man who *inter alia* put a cat in a gas oven, hanged a puppy in the garage and threatened his wife with a knife, Lawton L.J. said the words "mental illness"

> "are ordinary words of the English language. They have no particular medical significance. They have no particular legal significance . . . . Ordinary words of the English language should be construed in the way that ordinary sensible people would construe them . . . . I ask myself, what would the ordinary sensible person have said about the patient's condition in this case if he had been informed of his behaviour to the dogs, the cat and his wife. In my judgment such a person would have said 'Well, the fellow is obviously mentally ill.' "

This robust approach will appeal to some but it amounts to no more than a classification based upon behaviour. Further, an admission that the words have neither medical nor legal significance plays into the hands of critics of psychiatry such as Szasz and Laing. To Szasz "mental illness is a metaphor" used to cover people who are "socially deviant or inept, or in conflict with individuals, groups or institutions" (1973, p. 114).

Secondly, there is *severe mental impairment*. This concept replaces severe subnormalities. *Severe mental impairment* is defined as "a state of arrested or incomplete development of mind (not amounting to severe mental impairment) which includes significant impairment of intelligence and social functioning and is associated with abnormally aggressive or seriously irresponsible conduct on the part of the person concerned" (M.H.A. 1983, s.1(2)). "Impairment" is the term used by the World Health Organisation in its *International Classification of Impairments, Disabilities and Handicap*, to describe any loss or abnormality of psychological, physiological or anatomical structure or function. Concern may be expressed about the words "is associated with" for it appears that the test might be satisfied by demonstrating an event in the patient's past. The Minister of Health has said that "a patient's past conduct may be highly relevant as evidence . . . for those who must appraise his conduct and state of mind" (*H.C. Special Standing Committee*, May 11, 1982).

There are also two minor categories of mental disorder. *Mental impairment* is defined in the same way as severe impairment, except that it includes "significant," as opposed to "severe" impairment of intelligence and social functioning. It is not at all clear what the difference is between "severe" and "significant" impairment. It reflects "only a subtle difference in emphasis" (*Gostin*, 1982, p. 1129).

The legal effect of replacing the term "subnormality" by "mental impairment" is to remove most *mentally handicapped* people from the provisions of mental health legislation. A government spokesman said the intention behind the definitions of "mental impairment" and "severe mental impairment" is to limit the effect of the mental health legislation on mentally handicapped people "to those very few people for whom detention is essential so that treatment can be provided and for whom detention in prison should be avoided" (Lord Elton, H.L. Vol. 426, col. 533). But, since the definition of mental disorder in section 4(1) of the 1959 Act, which includes those who are suffering from "arrested or incomplete development of mind" was not amended by the 1982 Act, *mentally handicapped* people may continue to be subject to provisions which require the person only to be suffering from mental disorder. Such persons, therefore, remain liable to detention under the provisions of sections 2 and 4 of the 1983 Act (see below). They may also come within the jurisdiction of the Court of Protection (see below).

The second minor category of mental disorder is *psychopathic disorder*. This is defined (M.H.A. 1959, s.4(4), as amended by M.H.(A.)A. 1982, s.2(2): see now M.H.A. 1983, s.1(2)) as "a persistent disorder or disability of mind (whether or not including a significant impairment of intelligence) which results in abnormally aggressive or seriously irresponsible conduct on the part of the person concerned." The requirement in the 1959 Act that the disorder required or was susceptible to medical treatment has been removed but section 3(2)(*b*) of the 1983 Act incorporates in the provision relating to admission for treatment that "in the case of psychopathic disorder or mental impairment, that such treatment is likely to alleviate or prevent a deterioration of his condition."

It will have been observed that "mental illness" apart, the three forms of mental disorder all refer to "abnormally aggressive or seriously irresponsible conduct." They all may also include impairment of intelligence. The three are thus similar in scope and objective. They are also tautological, as Gostin notes, "in that they infer a disease from anti-social behaviour, while purporting to explain that behaviour by a disease" (1982, p. 1127).

It remains for us to consider what is meant by the expression in section 1(2) of the 1983 Act "any other disorder or disability of mind." The scope of this is heavily dependent upon the scope of "mental illness" and, to a lesser extent, of "psychopathic disorder." In Parliament in 1959, the examples were given of brain damage resulting from an injury or a physical disease such as *encephalitis*. Yet in many cases the results of such damage will be classified as mental illness or psychopathic disorder. Hoggett believes that neuroses and personality disorders fall to be classified in this residuary category unless they result in abnormally aggressive or seriously irresponsible behavior (1976, p. 50). If a person's disorder only fits within this residuary category, he cannot be made the subject of a hospital or guardianship order, or be admitted for treatment under section 3 of the 1983 Act or received into guardianship under section 7(2) of the 1983 Act, but he can be compulsorily admitted for observation under sections 2 or 3 of the 1983 Act or taken to a place of safety under sections 135 or 136 of that Act.

II. *Informal Admission and Holding Powers*

Most admissions to mental illness hospitals and units are informal (this word is preferable to "voluntary" for reasons that will become apparent). *Ninety per cent.* of admissions in 1980 were informal. Gostin in *A Human Condition* (1975, p. 16) states that "there is no genuinely voluntary action unless the informal patient has a free choice among alternatives." There may not be any alternatives or the patient may not know of alternatives or be told of them. Further, "demonstrated failures to train patients adequately for greater autonomy and adaptation to non-standardized community living may effectively prevent the institutionalized resident from returning to society" (*idem.* see also *E. Goffman*, 1961). It may also be asked how many patients understand informal status. Nor should it be overlooked that many enter hospital "voluntarily" because they fear that if they do not they will be compulsorily detained.

Informal admissions are governed by section 131 of the 1983 Act. In principle this provides for patients to enter a mental hospital as they would enter any other hospital. Secondly, a patient, who was compulsorily detained, may choose at the end of his detention to remain in mental hospital informally. Parents can arrange for the informal admission of a child under 16. A child between 16 and 18, who is capable of expressing his wishes, can make his own arrangements without his parents' consent (M.H.A. 1983, s.131(2)). Until a child is 16, any request for discharge must be made by the parent. Until the coming into operation of the 1982 Act there was no independent means of review of a parent's actions. But section 41 of the 1982 Act gave patients under the age of 16 the right to apply to a mental health review tribunal. In addition there is a duty on hospital managers to refer to a tribunal any patient under the age of 16 who has been detained for one year without a tribunal hearing (M.H.A. 1983, s.68(2)).

The informal patient is free to leave the hospital, except where the provisions of section 5(2) of the 1983 Act are invoked. This provides that if the medical practitioner in charge of the treatment of the patient considers that an application for formal admission should be made, he can make a written report to the hospital managers to this effect, stating that it appears that an application for admission for observation or treatment ought to be made. The patient can then be detained for a period of up to 72 hours from the time when "the report is so furnished." The medical practitioner in charge of the treatment of a patient in a hospital may nominate one other medical practitioner on the staff of the hospital to act for him in his absence for the purposes of section 5 (M.H.A. 1983, s.5(3)). The provision legitimising an application in respect of a patient already in hospital is couched in very wide terms. There seems to be no reason why it should not be used to detain a patient who has entered hospital for treatment for a physical complaint. But the provision is not greatly used. "Medical practitioner" is not further defined, nor does the Act amplify what is meant by "in charge of the treatment of a patient." It must be assumed that the Act intends these powers to be exercised by the consultant psychiatrist under whose care the patient has been admitted or is being treated, but it is not so stated.

The 1982 Act also provided additional holding powers for the first time. If it appears to a nurse of the "prescribed class" that an informal patient who is receiving treatment for mental disorder is suffering from mental disorder to such a degree that it is necessary for his health or safety or for the protection of others, for him to be immediately restrained from leaving the hospital and it is not practicable to secure the immediate attendance of a practitioner for the purpose of furnishing a report under section 5(2) of the 1983 Act (that is the medical practitioner in charge of treatment or the practitioner nominated by him), the nurse may record that fact in writing (s.5(4)). The report must be delivered by the nurse, or someone authorised by him, to the managers of the hospital as soon as possible after it is made (M.H.A. 1983, s.5(5)). The patient may then be detained in the hospital for a period of six hours from the time when that fact is so recorded or until the earlier arrival of the medical practitioner in charge of treatment or his nominated practitioner (M.H.A. 1983, s.5(4)). There is no power to renew this period. Only those nurses "prescribed" by an order of the Secretary of State have this authority. It is to be expected that registered mental nurses and registered nurses for the mentally handicapped will be prescribed (see *DHSS*, 1981, para. 22). Since the power to detain comes into effect only when the record is made, a nurse will have to rely on common law powers or section 3(1) of the Criminal Law Act 1967 for the period between detention of a patient threatening a dangerous act and the making of the record.

III. *Compulsory Admission for a Period not exceeding 72 Hours*

The 1983 Act authorises compulsory detention of patients for a period not to exceed 72 hours in a number of different contexts. (For a discussion of why compulsory powers are used see *Dawson*, 1972).

(a) Detention by police (M.H.A. 1983, s.136)

Any police officer may remove to a "place of safety" any person whom he finds in a "place to which the public has access" and who appears to be suffering from mental disorder and to be in need of immediate care or control, provided the police officer thinks removal to a place of safety is necessary in the interests of that person or for the protection of other persons. This power can be used even where the person involved has committed no criminal offence and the police officer has no power of arrest. No magistrate's warrant is required and medical evidence need not be produced. Once at the place of safety (in practice usually a police station or hospital), the person may be detained for up to 72 hours "for the purpose of enabling him to be examined by a medical practitioner and to be interviewed by an approved social worker and of making any necessary arrangements for his treatment or care" (M.H.A., 1983, s.136(2)).

The provision is widely used (there were 1,623 cases in 1979) and, though apparently it is not abused (see *Rollin*, 1969 and *Walker and McCabe*, 1973, *cf. Gostin*, 1975, p. 31), it is capable of abuse. The absence of procedural safeguards should cause concern. Section 136 is based on the assumption that the police are capable of diagnosing mental disorder and deciding whether treatment is necessary. There is no evidence that they are and it would surprise many, if given their education, training and experience, they had any insight into the problem at all. Whitehead (1974) finds it odd that any police constable can remove a person to a police station when experienced social workers cannot remove a patient to a hospital without the opinion of a doctor.

The case of *Carter* v. *Commissioner of the Police for the Metropolis* (1975) shows how section 136 may be used. A woman, with no history of mental illness, was taken from outside her own flat to a police station and later to a mental hospital. Her attempt to sue the police for false imprisonment did not succeed. The doctor at the hospital to which she was taken decided she was not in need of treatment and neither the courts nor the police investigated whether her actions posed a danger to herself or others. The police version of the story was that she was shouting abuse: hers that she was standing calmly in her doorway. Unfortunately, whether section 136 existed or not, the police would have detained her. There is no doubt that they could have claimed she was committing a whole gamut of offences (causing a breach of the peace; obstructing a police officer; insulting behaviour, etc.). There is, however, greater control of police powers in these contexts than in connection with section 136.

(b) Detention under warrant (M.H.A. 1983, s.135)

An approved social worker may lay an information on oath to a magistrate for the area where the patient is (this can be done at any time and in any place where a magistrate is available). The information must state that there is reasonable cause to suspect that a person believed to be suffering from mental disorder either (a) has been or is being ill-treated, neglected or kept otherwise than under proper control or (b) being unable to care for himself if living alone. The magistrate may then issue a warrant, which need not name the patient (s.135(5)). It must, however, specify the place where he is. The warrant is addressed to any police officer who must, in executing it, be accompanied by an approved social worker and a doctor (s.134(5)). The warrant authorises entry, if need be by force, and the removal to a place of safety of the patient, if this is thought fit. An application can then be made under Part II of the 1983 Act (see below) or other arrangements may be made for the patient's treatment or care. The patient may be detained in a place of safety for up to 72 hours (s.135(3)).

The provision is designed to protect patients whose families for whatever reason are not looking after them adequately. It is also used in the case of patients living alone who barricade themselves in and refuse all offers of assistance. Section 135 is little used (only 10 cases in 1979).

A place of safety is defined as residential accommodation provided by a local social services department under Part III of the National Assistance Act 1948 or Schedule 2, para. 8 of the National Health Service Act 1977, a hospital as defined by the 1983 Act (s.145(1)), a police station, a mental nursing home (see s.21 of Registered Homes Act 1984), a residential home for mentally disordered persons or "any other suitable place the occupier of which is willing temporarily to receive the patient" (M.H.A. 1983, s.135(6)).

(c) Emergency admission for assessment (M.H.A. 1983, s.4)

This is the simplest form of admission and, not surprisingly, has become the most common. Thus, in 1979 8,398 persons were admitted under the old section 29 (this is less than half the number in 1970). This accounted for 60 per cent. of the total number of short-term compulsory admissions in that year (*Gostin*, 1975, p. 28). According to Enoch and Barker (1965) many hospitals were receiving over 80 per cent. of compulsory patients through section 29 and Harbert (1965) reports that in some local authorities over 90 per cent. of compulsory admissions were "urgent." There are, however, marked regional variations.

It is important to realise that, as Gostin (1975, p. 29) puts it:

> "the act of compulsory admission . . . may be more traumatic than any subsequent detention. Furthermore, modern treatments and factors of inertia within hospitals often render a patient willing to accept the situation soon after compulsory admission; and, of course, factors of inertia increase the longer the patient remains in hospital."

There have been fears expressed that, what was then, section 29 is misused (*Ball*, 1967; *Harbert*, 1965; *BASW*, 1974; *Gostin*, 1975). Its over-use (and misuse) may be attributable to the resentment that GP's feel over the delay involved in applications under sections 2 or 3. Section 4 should only be used in "real emergencies" (*Percy*, 1957, para. 409). Evidence suggests that at present that is far from the case.

The procedure under the old section 29 was tightened up by the 1982 Amendment Act (s.3(3), (4)). The criteria for an application are now that it is of "urgent necessity" that the person be admitted to hospital and that compliance with the full procedure for admission for assessment under section 2 would involve "undesirable delay." (M.H.A. 1983, s.4(2)). The application may be made either by an approved social worker or the nearest relative of the patient. The meaning of "nearest relative" is to be found in section 26 of the 1983 Act.

"Relative" means one of the following, and "nearest relative" means whoever comes first on the list, ignoring people not ordinarily resident in the United Kingdom and people under the age of 18 unless married to the patient (s.26 of the 1983 Act). The list is:

(a) husband or wife: the spouse comes first even if he or she is under 18. The spouse can be disregarded if the couple are permanently separated by court order or by agreement or if one of them is in desertion of the other (s.26(5)(*b*)). If the patient is unmarried or his spouse can be disregarded, a co-habitant of not less than 6 months' standing must be treated as his spouse (M.H.A. 1983, s.26(6)).

(b) son or daughter: this includes adopted children, but not step-children or a man's illegitimate children (M.H.A. 1983, s.26(2)). If there are several children, the eldest is preferred, irrespective of sex.

(c) father or mother (M.H.A. 1983, s.26(1)(*c*)): the father formerly took precedence over the mother, but no longer does so (the change was made by M.H.(A.)A. 1982, s.14(2)). If the child is in care under a care order or parental rights have been assumed by resolution in respect of a child in voluntary care, the local authority takes the place of the parent concerned (see M.H.A. 1983, s.27, Child Care Act 1980, ss.3 and 10(2)). If the child is a ward of court, no application can be made without the court's consent and the functions of the nearest relative can only be exercised with its leave (M.H.A. 1983, s.33).

(d) brother or sister

(e) grandparent

(f) grandchild
(g) uncle or aunt
(h) nephew or niece.

Within categories (d) to (h) the same principles apply. If no one comes within any of these categories, there is no "relative" or "nearest relative."

It is provided that where someone "ordinarily resides with or is cared for by one or more of his relatives (or, if he is for the time being an in-patient in a hospital, he last ordinarily resided or was cared for by one or more of his relatives)" that person shall be his nearest relative (s.26(4)). If there are two or more such persons, full-blooded relatives are preferred to half-blooded, and the elder or eldest is to be preferred, irrespective of sex (s.26(3)). It is important to note that a prospective patient may be "cared for" by a relative even if the two do not share a residence.

The 1982 Act also added to the list "a person other than a relative, with whom the patient ordinarily resides" (or ordinarily resided prior to admission to hospital) and "with whom he has or had been ordinarily residing" for not less than five years. Such a person is to be treated as if he came last on the hierarchy of relatives listed in section 26(1) of the 1983 Act (s.26(7)). As a result of these recent changes in the law, this person could become the patient's nearest relative. It is further provided that such a person is not to displace the spouse of a married patient, unless the spouse is to be "disregarded" (s.26(7)(*b*)) (as to this see the discussion of s.26(5)(*b*) above).

An application for admission under section 4 must be accompanied by a medical recommendation complying with section 2 of the 1983 Act; if "practicable," this must be by a practitioner who has previous acquaintance with the patient (s.4(3)). No application can be made unless the applicant has personally seen the patient within the previous 24 hours (M.H.A. 1983, ss.11(5), 4(5)).

A patient must be admitted to hospital within 24 hours beginning from the time he is medically examined or when the application is made, whichever is the earlier (M.H.A. 1959, s.31(1)(*b*), as amended by M.H.(Amend.)A. 1982, s.3(4)(*a*)). Once admitted to hospital, the patient can only be detained under a section 4 application for up to 72 hours from the time he was admitted. The admission can be converted into one under section 25 (below), if within those 72 hours a second medical recommendation is received by the managers (this must comply with the requirements of section 28 (below). If this is done, the authority to detain is extended to 28 days beginning with the day of the patient's admission under section 29.

IV. *Admission for Assessment (28 days)*

Section 2 of the 1983 Act provides the power to detain a person for up to 28 days for assessment, or assessment followed by treatment. The 1959 legislation (s.25) had provided for admission for "observation." The reason for the change is explained in the White Paper accompanying the 1982 Bill as follows:

> "Because of developments in psychiatry since the Act was passed the power in s.25 is now used also as a short-term treatment power. It is therefore felt that 'assessment' is a more suitable term than 'observation' as it implies more active intervention to form a diagnosis and to plan treatment." (*DHSS*, 1981, para. 17).

An application for admission for assessment may be made on the grounds that the patient is:
- (a) suffering from mental disorder of a nature or degree which warrants his detention in hospital "for assessment (or for assessment followed by medical treatment)"; and
- (b) he ought to be so detained in the interests of his own health or safety or with a view to protection of others (M.H.A. 1983, s.2(2)).

The application must be made either by an approved social worker or the patient's nearest relative (s.11(1)). The applicant must have seen the patient within the period of 14 days ending with the date of the application (M.H.A. 1983, s.11(5)). If the application is made by an approved social worker, he must, before or within a reasonable time after an application is made, inform the nearest relative that an application is to be or has been made and of the power of the nearest relative to discharge the patient (M.H.A. 1983, ss.11(3) and 23(2)(*a*)). The 1982 Act gave the nearest relative this power for the first time. However, unlike the case of admission for treatment (below), there is no obligation on the approved social worker to consult with and obtain the agreement of the nearest relative prior to making an application for assessment.

An admission for assessment must be founded on and accompanied by the written recommendations of two medical practitioners, one of whom must have been approved by the Secretary of State as having special experience in the diagnosis or treatment of mental disorder (M.H.A. 1983, s.2(3)). The two medical practitioners must have examined the patient either together or within five days of each other (M.H.A. 1983, s. 12(1)). Only one recommendation can come from a practitioner on the staff of the hospital to which the patient is to be admitted (M.H.A. 1983, s.12(3)), except where compliance with this requirement would result in "delay involving serious risk to the health or safety of the patient" *and* one of the practitioners giving the recommendations spends less than half of his time in Health Service employment at the hospital (*and*, where one of the practitioners is a consultant, the other does not work in a grade in which he is under that consultant's directions) (M.H.A. 1983, s.12(4)(*c*)). A practitioner is precluded from making a recommendation if he is, or is related to, a person who receives or has an interest in the receipt of any payments made on account of the maintenance of the patient (M.H.A. 1983, s.12(5)(*d*)). Nor may the doctor be on the staff of the admitting hospital or mental nursing home or be related to one who is (M.H.A. 1983, s.12(5)(*e*)): part-time practitioners are exempted from this (M.H.A. 1983, s.12(6)). Further, he cannot be the applicant (s.12(5)(*a*)) or the applicant's partner (s.12(5)(*b*)) or employed as an assistant by the applicant (s.12(5)(*c*)) and he cannot himself be related to the patient.

A patient admitted to hospital may be detained for a period not to exceed 28 days (M.H.A. 1983, s.2(4)). It is clear from the change in wording that treatment may be undertaken. As Gostin notes (1982, p. 1129): "this may suggest that, apart from the period of detention, there may be very little difference between an admission for assessment and for treatment."

The 1982 Act gave patients admitted for assessment the right to apply to a Mental Health Review Tribunal within 14 days of being admitted. (see now M.H.A. 1983, s.66(1)(*a*), (2)(*a*)). The White Paper accompanying the 1982 Bill says that the Tribunal "will usually have to rely largely on the medical and social workers' reports made at the time of admission, with perhaps an oral report from the patient's responsible medical officer" (1981, para. 18). It seems that a responsible medical officer will be able to continue with the treatment of a patient detained under section 2 even after the patient has exercised his right to apply to a Tribunal.

V. *Admission for Treatment (six months)*

An application for admission for treatment may be made on the grounds that the patient is:

(a) suffering from one of the four categories of mental disorder (above) of a nature or degree which warrants the detention of the patient in hospital for medical treatment *and*

(b) in the case of psychopathic disorder or mental impairment that such treatment is likely to alleviate or prevent a deterioration of his condition *and*

(c) it is necessary for the health or safety of the patient or for the protection of other persons that he should receive such treatment and that it cannot be provided unless he is compulsorily admitted for treatment (M.H.A. 1983, s.3(1)).

The "treatability" test only applies to psychopathic disorder and mental impairment and not therefore to the other categories of mental disorder. So, mentally ill people and those with severe mental impairment may be admitted under section 3 when they are unlikely to benefit from treatment in the sense that their condition may not improve: "these people might nevertheless need to be admitted on occasions, for example, to tide them over a crisis" (*DHSS*, 1978, para. 2.40). However, if the responsible medical officer reclassifies a detained patient from mental illness or severe mental impairment to either psychopathic disorder or mental impairment, and makes a report to that effect under section 16(1) of the 1983 Act, the authority to detain the patient terminates unless the patient's consultant certifies that further medical treatment in hospital is likely to alleviate or prevent a deterioration of the patient's condition (M.H.A. 1983, s.16(2)). Before reclassifying a patient, the responsible medical officer must consult one or more persons who have been professionally concerned with the patient's treatment (M.H.A. 1983, s.16(3)). The Act does not state what "consult" means. It is to be expected that the Mental Health Act Commission (below) will issue guidance on this.

Patients admitted for treatment may be detained for a period not to exceed six months. The authority for detention may be renewed for a further period of six months and subsequently for periods of one year at a time (M.H.A. 1983, s.20). The authority for detention may be renewed if the responsible medical officer furnishes a report to the hospital managers stating that the original grounds of admission still apply (M.H.A. 1983, s.20(3)(4)). The treatability criterion applies to cases of renewal, except that in the case of mental illness or severe mental impairment it is an alternative that the patient "if discharged, is unlikely to be able to care for himself, obtain the care which he needs or to guard himself against serious exploitation" (M.H.A. 1983, s.20(4)). We are told that few cases can be expected where detention is necessary but where there can be little expectation of treatment having beneficial effect (*DHSS*, 1978, para. 2.44). Before furnishing a report renewing the detention of a patient, the responsible medical officer must consult one or more persons who have been professionally concerned with the patient's medical treatment (M.H.A. 1983, s.20(5)). Where a report has been furnished, the patient has the right to apply to a Mental Health Review Tribunal. (M.H.A. 1983, s.66(1)(*f*)).

An application for admission for treatment may be made either by the patient's nearest relative (for definition of this see above) or by an approved social worker. (M.H.A. 1983, s.11(1)). The approved social worker must, if practicable, consult the nearest relative before making an application, (M.H.A. 1983, s.11(4)). The nearest relative need not give express consent, but if he notifies the approved social worker or the local social services authority that he objects, the application cannot be made (M.H.A. 1983, s.11(4)). If the nearest relative objects unreasonably to admission, an approved social worker or other specified persons can apply to the county court for an order appointing him or any other proper person to act in place of the nearest relative (M.H.A. 1983, s.29(1), (2)). The county court may specify a period for which such an order will remain in force (M.H.A. 1983, s.29(5)).

The application for admission for treatment must have the support of two medical recommendations (M.H.A. 1983, s.3(3)). These must comply with the same requirements as govern admission for assessment (above). In addition, a medical recommendation for admission for treatment must state the specific grounds for the doctor's opinion, specifying whether other methods of dealing with the patient exist and, if they do, why they are not appropriate. (M.H.A. 1983, s.3(3)(*b*)). The importance of this is that it forces doctors to think of hospitalisation as a last resort.

VI. *Reception into Guardianship (six months)*

A patient of 16 or over may be received into guardianship on the grounds that:

(a) he is suffering from one of the four specific forms of mental disorder (above) of a nature or degree which warrants his reception into guardianship; and

(b) this is necessary in the interests of the welfare of the patient or for the protection of others (M.H.A. 1983, s.7(1), (2)).

Children under 16 cannot be received into guardianship, though care proceedings may be brought under section 1 of the Children and Young Persons Act 1969 if a ground exists (possibly "moral danger" under s.1(2)(*c*)) *and* the child is in need of "care or control which he is unlikely to receive unless the court makes an order." A care order or supervision order or hospital or guardianship order could then be made (see s.1(3)(*b*)(*c*)(*d*)(*e*)). See above.

The procedures for reception into guardianship are the same as for an admission for treatment. Provisions governing duration of guardianship follow those for admission for treatment (see M.H.A. 1983, s.20). The maximum period is six months, unless it is renewed, as it may be, initially for another six months and then for periods of a year at a time (s.20(2)).

The person named as guardian in the application must either be a local social services authority or a private individual approved by the authority (M.H.A. 1983, s.7(5)). The guardian may be the applicant himself. If a private individual is to act as guardian, the application must be accompanied by a statement in writing by that person that he is willing to act. The guardian has the following powers:

(a) power to require the patient to reside at a place specified by the authority or person named as guardian;

(b) power to require the patient to attend at places and times so specified for the purpose of medical treatment, occupation, education or training;

(c) power to require access to the patient to be given, at a place where the patient is residing, to any medical practitioner, approved social worker or other person so specified (M.H.A. 1983, s.8).

Previous legislation did not define powers: it merely gave the guardian the powers that a father has over a child under 14 and these are far from clear (*Eekelaar*, 1973).

The 1983 Act (s.9(1)(*a*)) empowers the Secretary of State to make regulations to govern the guardian's exercise of his powers but the opportunity to do this in the Mental Health (Hospital, Guardianship and Consent to Treatment) Regulations 1983 was not taken. It is accordingly difficult to see what courses of action are open to the guardian should the patient refuse, for example, to reside in a particular place. The 1983 Regulations do, however, set out the duties of a private guardian (that is, as opposed to a local authority guardianship) (see reg. 12). The duties are:

(i) to appoint a registered medical practitioner to act as the nominated attendant of the patient;

(ii) to notify the responsible local social services authority of the name and address of the nominated medical attendant;

(iii) in exercising powers and duties conferred or imposed on him by the 1983 Act or 1983 Regulations, to comply with such directions as the authority may give;

(iv) to furnish the authority with all such reports or other information with regard to the patient as the authority may from time to time require;

(v) to notify the authority—

(a) on the reception of the patient into guardianship, of his address and the address of the patient, and

(b) of any permanent change of either address;

(vi) if the permanent change of address is in the area of a different authority, to notify that authority and tell the authority previously responsible;

(vii) in the event of the death of the patient, or termination of the guardianship by discharge, transfer or otherwise, to notify the responsible authority as soon as reasonably practicable.

Guardianship is little used. The Butler Committee (1975) recommended it should be used more frequently by the courts when dealing with offenders who do not need hospital treatment. There is, however, no evidence that this is happening.

7. The Legal Status of Mental Patients

In the past legislation has had little to say about the rights or welfare of mental patients whilst in hospital. The law regulated the admission to mental hospital and provided for departure from such institutions but it said very little about the legal status of the patient. The domain of the clinical relationship between the medical staff and the patient was a veritable legal Alsatia into which the King's writ did not run. The law's lack of concern for the rights of psychiatric patients was attacked in the Mind study, *A Human Condition* (1975). To a large degree as a result of this publication there was a shift of policy in the 1982 Act. This (see now the 1983 Act) contains detailed regulations relating to the rights of detained patients to consent to treatment. It establishes the Mental Health Act Commission which is given general oversight of conditions of detention of patients. It also makes provision for after-care of patients. (See Chap. 8).

I. *Consent to Treatment*

The legal position under the 1959 Act regarding a detained patient's right to refuse treatment was not clear. It was the Department of Health and Social Security's view that, where the purpose of the detention was treatment, the 1959 Act gave the responsible medical officers implied authority to treat a patient, even against that patient's wishes. This view was doubted by Jacob (1976), Gostin (1979, 1981) and by the Confederation of Health Service Employees (1977). Part VI of the 1982 Act has removed any doubt by defining the extent to which treatment for mental disorder can be imposed. The consent provisions in the new law (now part IV of the Mental Health Act 1983) apply to any patient liable to be detained under the Mental Health Acts except (see M.H.A. 1983, s.56):

 (i) a patient who is liable to be detained by virtue of an emergency application and in respect of whom the second medical recommendation referred to in section 4(4)(*a*) has not been given and received;

 (ii) a patient who is liable to be detained by a doctor's or nurse's holding power (M.H.A. 1983, s.5(2) and s.5(4)), or police power (M.H.A. 1983, s.136) or by removal by warrant (M.H.A. 1983, s.135), or who is being detained in a place of safety pursuant to a hospital order (M.H.A. 1983, s.37(4));

 (iii) a patient who has been conditionally discharged and has not been recalled to hospital (M.H.A. 1983, s.42(2); see also ss.73 and 74);

 (iv) a patient who has been remanded to hospital for report (M.H.A. 1983, s.35).

Guardianship patients and informal patients are not, of course, "liable to be detained" but they are protected in the case of the most serious treatments (those requiring consent *and* a second opinion) (s.56(2)).

The phrase "liable to be detained" includes those on authorised leaves of absence under section 17 of the 1983 Act.

A patient who is excluded from the consent to treatment provisions of Part IV of the 1983 Act is to be viewed as if he were an informal psychiatric patient or an ordinary patient receiving treatment for a physical ailment. He is, therefore, subject to the ordinary principles of the common law and these usually (*cf. Skegg* 1974) require a legally effective consent to medical treatment. Exceptions are made in cases of necessity (*Skegg*, 1974). The 1983 Act's framework embraces only medical treatment for mental disorders. It does not apply to treatment for physical disorders. Nor would it apply to operations of a non-therapeutic nature such as a vasectomy or an abortion. It is not clear when such treatment may be given to a mentally incompetent person who cannot give a legally effective consent. Skegg argues that "if the patient is likely to be permanently incapable of consenting and no one is authorised to consent on his behalf, a doctor should be justified in doing whatever good medical practice dictates should be done in the patient's interests" (1974). As far as therapeutic treatments for physical disorders are concerned, this is a readily defensible position. It may be more difficult to support outside such a context. As Gostin (1982) notes, "the legal responsibility of the doctor . . . becomes more uncertain where the patient is non-volitional or non-objecting, as opposed to expressly refusing consent."

The 1983 Act distinguishes between two types of medical treatment for mental disorder: (i) treatment requiring consent *and* a second opinion (s.57); (ii) treatment requiring consent *or* a second opinion (s.58). Treatment for mental disorder given by or under the direction of the responsible medical officer which does not come within either of these categories does not require the consent of the patient (s.63). The Minister of Health's defence of this is to the effect that: "hospitals are places of treatment and we cannot have hospitals in which people are locked up and left to wander about without receiving treatment" (*Special Standing Committee*, June 29, 1982).

(a) Treatment requiring consent and a second opinion

Surgical operations for destroying brain tissue or for destroying the functioning of brain tissue (psychosurgery) and such other forms of treatment as may be specified by regulations made by the Secretary of State for Health and Social Services require consent *and* a second opinion (s.57(1)). The only form of treatment as yet specified is the surgical implantation of hormones for the purpose of reducing male sexual drive (see Mental Health (Hospital, Guardianship and Consent to Treatment) Regulations 1983 (S.I. 1983 No. 893, reg.16(1)(*a*)).

It is to be hoped that other serious treatments that are irreversible or drastic will be provided for under this section (the Minister of Health's statement, H.C. Deb., Vol. 29, col. 80 gives some indication of likely inclusions). Before regulations are made concerned bodies must be consulted (M.H.A. 1983, s.57(4)). It is, however, psychosurgery which has caused greatest concern. Between 1979 and 1982, 207 psychosurgical operations on informal patients and four on detained patients were carried out in England and Wales (see *Special Standing Committee*, June 29, 1982). Psychosurgery involves an irreversible lesion in structurally normal brain tissue. Doubt has been expressed as to whether it is always administered in the most appropriate circumstances (*Gostin*, 1982 (*b*)).

In recognition of the seriousness of psychosurgery (and some other as yet unspecified treatments) section 57 departs from a fundamental common law principle by requiring a second opinion in addition to the consent of the patient. The second opinion must be given by a medical practitioner, not being the responsible medical officer, and two other persons, not being doctors, each of whom are to be appointed by the Secretary of State. The three persons must certify in writing that, having regard to the likelihood of the treatment alleviating or preventing a deterioration of the patient's condition, the treatment should be gven (s.57(2)). Before giving a certificate, the medical practitioner must consult two other persons who have been professionally concerned with the patient's medical treatment, one of whom is a nurse and the other of whom is neither a nurse nor a medical practitioner (s.57(3)). The latter might be a social worker, a psychologist or occupational therapist. It is important to note that a medical practitioner cannot give a certificate if no other professionals, apart from nurses, have been involved in the patient's treatment.

Section 57 extends to informal patients as well (s.56(2)). It does not, however, apply to patients detained for 72 hours or remanded for reports or to conditionally discharged patients who are liable to recall. In these cases consent is required but a second opinion is not. This was an unfortunate, and probably unintended, gap in the 1982 Act. It remains in the 1983 Act.

(b) Treatment requiring consent or a second opinion

Section 58 of the 1983 Act provides for certain types of treatment to require *either* the consent of the patient *or* a second opinion. These are (*a*) treatments specified by the Secretary of State in regulations and (*b*) the administration of medicine by any means (not being a treatment specified in (*a*) or in s.57). As far as (*a*) is concerned, the Government has specified electro-convulsive therapy (E.C.T.) as the form of treatment to which this section applies (see S.I. 1983 No. 893, reg.16(2)(*a*)). The reason why the section does not specifically include E.C.T. is that as practice developed, a future Secretary of State might wish to "promote it or relegate it from one division to another" (*per* Minister of

Health, H.C. Deb., Vol. 29, col. 86). Section 58 applies to category (*b*) treatments only if three months or more have elapsed since the first occasion during the period of detention when medication was "administered by any means" for the patient's mental disorder. The Secretary of State may by order vary the length of this period M.H.A. 1983 (s.58(2)).

The "three month rule" is intended to give the psychiatrist time to consider a treatment programme which suits the patient. It has been said (by the Under Secretary of State) to be "long enough to allow a proper valuation and assessment of what, if any, long term treatment may be needed" and to be "short enough to ensure that patients' consent, or a second opinion, is obtained before a long term course of drug treatment gets too far ahead" (*Special Standing Committee*, June 29, 1982).

The scheme provided for by section 58 envisages that a particular medication may fall into any of three conceptual categories, depending in each case upon whether it is considered hazardous, irreversible or not fully established: (i) it could be included in regulations or the code of practice for treatments requiring consent *and* a second opinion; (ii) it could be included in regulations for treatments requiring consent *or* a second opinion, in which case the "three month rule" would not apply; or (iii) if it is not included in any regulations or the code it will be subject to the "three month rule."

Section 58 treatments cannot be given unless the patient consents *or* a second opinion is secured. "Valid consent implies the ability, given an explanation in simple terms, to understand the nature, purpose and effect of the proposed treatment" (Cmnd. 7320, para. 6.23). The consent must be confirmed by a certification in writing by either the responsible medical officer or a medical practitioner appointed by the Secretary of State to the effect that the patient is capable of understanding the nature, purpose and likely effects and has consented to it (s.58(3)(*a*)). The second opinion must be given by a medical practitioner appointed by the Secretary of State, not being the responsible medical officer, who must certify in writing that the patient is not capable of understanding the nature, purpose and likely effects of the treatment or has not consented to it but that, having regard to the likelihood of its alleviating or preventing a deterioration of his condition, the treatment should be given (s.58(3)(*b*)). Before giving a certificate, the medical practitioner is required to consult two other persons who have been professionally concerned with the patient's medical treatment, one of whom is a nurse and the other is neither a nurse nor a medical practitioner. The Minister of Health has said that it would probably be very unusual for the psychiatrist who gives a certificate under paragraph (*b*) to give an open-ended opinion which would allow the treatment to go on for years. Rather, it was said, most psychiatrists would be likely to suggest that a course of treatment should be tried for a finite period (*Special Standing Committee*, June 29, 1982). The patient's protection lies in the responsible medical officer's obligation to furnish reports to the Secretary of State on the treatment and the patient's condition and in the powers of the Mental Health Act Commission (below, p.174).

The significance of section 58 must not be underestimated. Whatever was the position at common law, the law now allows for treatment to be given to a patient who understands its nature, purpose and likely effects and who refuses to give his consent to such treatment. His will can be overriden where a psychiatrist believes he needs psychiatric treatment. "Need for treatment" is substituted for "competency" as the governing criterion.

(c) Withdrawal of consent

A patient may at any time before the completion of the treatment withdraw his consent. Where he does so, the treatment is then regarded as a separate form of treatment (Mental Health (Amendment) Act 1982, s.60(1)). A patient may also withdraw his consent to a treatment plan (s.60(2)). The withdrawal provision applies to informal patients as well (s.56(2)). If the patient's psychiatrist considers that the discontinuance of the treatment or of treatment under the plan would cause serious suffering to the patient, the treatment can be continued (see M.H.A. 1983, s.62(2)).

It would seem, though it is not entirely clear, that upon the withdrawal of consent to the administration of medication the "three month rule" (above, p.144) would apply as of the date of the withdrawal of the consent.

(d) Urgent treatment

Treatment under sections 57 or 58 can be given without the need for consent or a second opinion if it is urgent. Urgent treatment is treatment which is "immediately necessary" (a) to save a patient's life or (b) to prevent a "serious deterioration of his condition" or (c) to "alleviate serious suffering by the patient," or (d) is "immediately necessary and represents the minimum interference necessary to prevent the patient from behaving violently or being a danger to himself or to others." There are exceptions for treatments which are irreversible (in the case of (b) or irreversible or hazardous (in the case of (c) and (d) (s.62(1)). "Irreversible" is defined somewhat unhelpfully as having "unfavourable irreversible physical or psychological consequences" and "hazardous" is defined equally unhelpfully as entailing "significant physical hazard" (s.62(3)). An example of favourable irreversible treatment is the removal of a brain tumour or diseased thyroid. The responsible medical officer is allowed (by s.62(2)) to override the patient's withdrawal of consent until a second opinion can be obtained, if discontinuing the treatment (or until a second opinion can be obtained, if discontinuing the treatment (or treatment under the plan) would cause the patient serious suffering.

The provisions relating to urgent treatment apply to informal patients as well (s.56(2)).

(e) Plans of treatment

It is provided by section 59 of the 1983 Act that any consent or certificate given under sections 57 or 58 may relate to a plan of treatment under which the patient is to be given, whether within a specified period or otherwise, one or more forms of treatment. Psychiatrists may thus decide upon an individual treatment plan for each patient which would allow for flexibility and variation within the context of the treatment objectives. He can respond to the patient's reaction to particular drugs or dosages and variations within the limits of the treatment plan do not require a fresh consent or certificate under sections 57 or 58. A patient may withdraw his consent to a treatment plan (M.H.A. 1983, s.60(2)).

(f) Review of treatment

Provision is made for the periodic review of treatment which has been authorised by a second psychiatric opinion under section 57(2) or section 58(3)(*b*) of the 1983 Act on the treatment and the patient's condition (M.H.A. 1983, s.62(1)). The responsible medical officer must furnish a report to the Secretary of State at the time the authority for the patient's detention is renewed and at any other time required by the Secretary of State. It should be noted that the Secretary of State's functions under section 61 are to be carried out by the Mental Health Act Commission (see M.H.A. 1983, s.121(2)(*b*)). It is to be assumed that more frequent reviews will be required where the treatment is particularly controversial or where the second psychiatric opinion favours a more speedy review of treatment. The Mental Health Act Commission is also given power to give notice to the responsible medical officer directing that a certificate given by the second medical practitioner under section 57(2) or section 58(3)(*b*) shall cease to apply. The patient's psychiatrist could only then continue the treatment if a further certificate were obtained.

II. *Access to the Courts*

Patients in mental hospitals do not enjoy open access to the courts of law of the land. This clear injustice is grounded in the fear that those suffering from mental disorder would use legal processes abusively or, at least, vexatiously. (See, for example, Lord Simon of Glaisdale in *Poultney* v. *Griffiths*, 1975). To institute proceedings mental patients must surmount a number of hurdles. Very few bother (there have been less than twenty actions since 1889, a statutory provision of that year is the earliest precursor to the current legislation). As Gostin notes, "These numbers may suggest that patients do not often exercise their right of access to the courts, and therefore that the provisions of section 141 [of the 1959 Act] (below, pp.148–149) are not necessary to protect hospital staff against unnecessary litigation" (1975). In response to widespread criticism and a finding by the European Commission of Human Rights in the *Ashingdane* case that section 141 infringed Article 6(1) of the European Convention which guarantees the right to a fair trial in the determination of a civil right (1982) (the case still awaits a decision from the Court on its merits), the 1982 Act effected a number of improvements and facilitated access to the courts by mental patients. Barriers, however, still exist.

Section 141 of the 1959 Act stated that except with the leave of the High Court, "no civil or criminal proceedings" were to be instituted against any person "in respect of any act purporting to be done in pursuance of" the Act of 1959. The High Court was not to give leave "unless satisfied that there [was] a substantial ground for the contention that the person to be proceeded against [had] acted in bad faith or without reasonable care." There were thus both procedural and substantive impediments.

The 1982 Act, s.60 (see now M.H.A. 1983, s.139) amended section 141 in three ways:

(i) in both civil and criminal cases, it removes the requirement that the person seeking leave to commence proceedings has to show that there are substantial grounds for the contention that the person to be proceeded against acted in bad faith or without reasonable care. It will, however, still be necessary to show bad faith or lack of reasonable care in the substantive proceedings;

(ii) the leave of the Director of Public Prosecutions (in Northern Ireland, the D.P.P. for Northern Ireland), not the High Court, is required before criminal proceedings can be brought against any person (the leave of the High Court is still required for civil proceedings); and

(iii) section 141 no longer applies to proceedings against the Secretary of State or against a health authority (as defined by the National Health Service Act 1977). See now M.H.A. 1983, s.139(4).

The third of these changes is the most significant since most of the proceedings that mental patients will want to bring will be against health authorities or the Secretary of State. But they will not all be. Section 141, as amended, will continue to apply to actions against other persons, for example social workers or the police. Such persons are not liable for any act purporting to be done in pursuance of the Mental Health Acts or of any rules or regulations made under them, whether on the ground of want of jurisdiction or on any other ground, unless the act was done in bad faith or without reasonable care (M.H.A. 1983, s.139(1)). An "act purporting to be done in pursuance of" the Acts covers any action, for example, a compulsory admission, where the defendant claims to be acting under authority granted by a particular provision of the Acts (or rules or regulations). Also, it has been held, somewhat dubiously, to apply to an allegation of assaulting a compulsory patient made against a nurse at Broadmoor (*Pountney* v.

Griffiths, 1975). Section 139(1) protects people who lacked the authority to act as they did, provided that what they did was in good faith and provided they took reasonable care. So, it would seem (see *Richardson* v. *London County Council*, 1957) that an honest mistake about the law can be a defence. But social workers, for example, will have little knowledge of the law (how much training in mental health legislation goes into an average C.Q.S.W. course?). How much effort can we, therefore, expect them to make to ensure that they do not make such mistakes? It was the view of two lawyer members of the Butler Committee (1975) that section 141 should have been amended to make it clear that the protection did not extend to mistakes of law. This has not been done.

Where acts relate to informal patients, section 139 applies, unless the acts are held not to be done "in pursuance of" the 1983 Act (as was the case in *R.* v. *Runighian*, 1977). There was an attempt in 1982 to exclude the provisions of section 141 in the case of informal patients but this was resisted by the Government on the ground that to do so would remove protection from someone who believed he was dealing with a detained patient (H.C. Deb., Vol. 29, col. 173). This is unconvincing for such a person would anyway be protected as he would be acting in good faith, unless, of course, he did not show reasonable care.

III. *Electoral Registration of Patients and Voting Rights*

Voting may only be exercised by those whose name appears on the register of electors as a resident of a particular locality. The Representation of the People Act 1949 (s.4(3)) does not allow a patient "in any establishment wholly or mainly for the reception and treatment of persons suffering from mental disorder" to use the hospital as a place of residence for voting purposes. The wording is odd and anomalies follow: an informal patient with a home address can register and vote; a patient in a psychiatric wing of a general hospital can also vote for the hospital may be used as place of residence for voting purposes. Two County Court actions brought by MIND in 1976 and 1981 (on the 1981 action, see *The Times*, September 17, 1981) established the principle that a resident of a mental illness or mental handicap hospital, who was not mentally disordered within the meaning of section 4 of the 1959 Act, could use the hospital as a place of residence for voting purposes. There followed circulars (R.P.A. 261 and H.N. (76) 180) giving hospitals and registration officers guidance.

The 1982 Act effected some reform on the question of registration and voting. It provides that informal patients should no longer be prevented from registering as electors solely because their only place of residence is a psychiatric hospital (M.H.(A.)A. 1982, s.62 and Sched. 2). Patients detained in hospital or a nursing home under the 1983 Act are not, accordingly, entitled to be registered as voters. A "voluntary mental patient" (the Act uses the word "voluntary") residing at a hospital can register to vote at the address at which he would be resident in the United Kingdom if he were not in hospital or any address at which he was residing in the United Kingdom, other than a mental hospital. To qualify he must make a declaration without any assistance (assistance does not include assistance necessitated by blindness or other physical incapacity). This must be attested in the prescribed manner (see Sched. 2). The declaration must specify the address outside the hospital at which the patient is to be registered as an elector. Once a patient's name is on the register he is entitled to apply for postal vote at election time. A patient is not allowed to use a mental hospital as a place of residence. It may have been thought that otherwise the result in a particular constituency might be materially affected by the existence of a large mental hospital within the constituency boundaries. The "no assistance" test does, as Gostin notes (1982), seemingly create an implicit "capacity test," apart from tests of incapacity existing at common law. This cannot be viewed as a desirable trend. (For a critical comment on the new provision see *Szasz*, 1982).

IV. *Correspondence of Patients*

Sections 36 and 134 of the 1959 Act gave the responsible medical officer the power under certain circumstances to withhold correspondence to or from both informal and detained patients. The 1982 Act replaced these much-criticised provisions by more limited powers, which apply moreover to detained patients only.

Section 134 of the 1982 Act authorises the hospital managers to withhold a detained patient's out-going mail from the Post Office, if the person to whom the packet is addressed requests by written notice that letters addressed to him should be stopped (s.134(1)). There are, in addition, powers to withhold post which are only applicable to patients in special hospitals (Broadmoor, Rampton, Park Lane, Moss Side). These apply where the hospital managers consider that the packet is "likely to cause distress to the person to whom it is addressed or to any other person (not being a person on the staff of the hospital) or to cause danger to any person" (s.134(1)(*b*)).

Further, the hospital managers may withhold post addressed to special hospital patients if, in their opinion, "it is necessary to do so in the interests of the safety of the patient or for the protection of other persons" (s.134(2)).

Hospital managers have the power to inspect and open any postal packet to determine whether its contents require it to be withheld under section 134 (s.134(4)).

Where post is withheld the hospital managers must record this (s.134(5)) (As to what must be recorded see S.I. 1983 No. 893, reg.17(2)), and give notice to the patient within seven days. In the case of packets addressed to special hospital patients withheld under section 134(2), notice must also be given to the person, if known, by whom the postal packet was sent. Persons who receive any such notice have six months to request the Mental Health Act Commission to review the decision to withhold post.

It is clear from the wording of section 134 that powers extend only to the withholding of post, or anything contained in a postal packet (s.134(4)). There is, accordingly, no authority to censor correspondence.

Section 134 does not apply to post to or from Ministers of the Crown, M.P.s, the Court of Protection, the Lord Chancellor's visitors, the Parliamentary Commissioner for Administration, the Health Service Commissioner for England or Wales or a local Commissioner, a Mental Health Review Tribunal, a Health Authority, local Social Services Authority, Community Health Council, Probation and After-Care Committee, the hospital managers where the patient is detained, any legally qualified person instructed by the patient to act as his legal adviser or the European Commission of Human Rights or the European Court of Human Rights. But any of these persons (or officials of these institutions) can request that communications addressed to them by the patient be withheld by the hospital managers under section 134(1)(*a*).

V. *Visitation Rights*

The psychiatric patient is also denied freedom of association. Limitations are placed on visits by friends and relatives which go beyond the "visiting hours" concept that we associate with general hospitals. The law, however, does give the patient some legal rights.

Thus: (i) an independent doctor authorised by the patient or his nearest relative must be permitted to visit the patient and examine him in private for the purpose of advising on an application to a Mental Health Review Tribunal or for the exercise of the relative's power of discharge (M.H.A. 1983, s.76(1)); (ii) the members of a Mental Health Review Tribunal must be allowed to interview the patient in private and the medical member to examine him and his records (Mental Health Review Tribunal Rules 1983, r.11) ((i) and (ii) only apply to detained patients); (iii) if the patient is in a mental nursing home, an inspector authorised by the DHSS must be allowed to visit and interview the patient in private, either to investigate any complaint about his treatment, or where there is reasonable cause to suspect lack of care. If the inspector is a doctor, he may examine the patient and his records (Registered Homes Act 1984, s.17); (iv) persons authorised by the independent bodies who have power to discharge patients in mental nursing homes must be allowed to visit and interview the patient and if the person is a doctor to examine the patient and his medical records (M.H.A. 1959, s.37(2) and (3)); (v) visitors appointed by the Lord Chancellor to assist the Court of Protection under section 102 of the 1983 Act may visit patients to investigate their legal capacity or provide other information needed by the Court to exercise its function of looking after the property and affairs of patients so disordered that they cannot do so themselves. If medically qualified, they may also examine the patient (s.103(6)). The reports are confidential (M.H.A. 1983, s.103(8)); (vi) the local authority social services department has a duty of visiting child patients over whom the authority has parental rights and powers (as a result of a care order or s.3 resolution) as well as patients subject to the authority's guardianship and patients over whom the authority acts as "nearest relative" (M.H.A. 1983, s.116).

VI. *Pocket Money*

Sickness and Invalidity Benefits, Widow's Benefit, and Retirement Pensions are subject to a reduction of two-fifths of the normal full benefit after the first eight weeks that a Health Service patient has been in hospital. After a year, there is a further reduction of two-fifths of the original, so that the patient is left with one-fifth of the full benefit to provide for extra comforts (National Health Service Act 1946, s.4). The Secretary of State for Health and Social Security may pay to patients such amounts as he thinks fit for their occasional personal expenses, where it appears that they would otherwise be without resources to meet those expenses (M.H.A. 1983, s.122(1)). If a patient has been receiving treatment continuously in hospital for not less than 52 weeks, and the responsible medical officer certifies that the patient is unable to appreciate the benefit payable, this may be stopped or reduced (National Insurance (Hospital In-patients) Amendment Regulations 1960).

VII. *Management of Property and Affairs*

Most of those who suffer from mental disorder are capable of managing their own affairs. The Court of Protection (it is an office, rather than a court) exists for those who cannot do so. The Court's jurisdiction arises "where, after considering the medical evidence" it is "satisfied that a person is incapable, by reason of mental disorder, of managing and administering his property and affairs" (M.H.A. 1983, s.94(2)). In an emergency the Court can act without making a formal determination of incapacity. It must have reason to believe that the person may be incapable, by reason of mental disorder, of managing and administering his property and affairs, and it must be of the opinion that it is necessary to make some immediate provision for matters within the court's powers (M.H.A. 1983, s.98). The need to go to the Court of Protection is most likely to arise where the patient has assets such as a business or investments which need to be managed or assets which need to be disposed of. The Court has, however, said (Leaflet

P.H. 1) that if a relative or friend, acting on the advice of the patient's doctor, thinks that in all the circumstances it would be in the patient's best interests to give up the tenancy of a rented home, it will raise no objection.

The Court's function is to "do or secure the doing of all such things as appear necessary or expedient" for the "maintenance or other benefit of the patient" or his family, or for providing for other people or purposes for which the patient might have been expected to provide were he not disordered, or for otherwise administering his affairs (M.H.A. 1983, s.95(1)). Section 96 of the 1983 Act contains a long list of things the Court may do. It includes the carrying out of any contract entered into by the patient, the dissolution of a partnership of which the patient is a member, buying and selling property, conducting legal proceedings, making a will. The list is much fuller than this and is not exhaustive. Once the patient becomes subject to the Court's jurisdiction, it has exclusive control over all his property and all his affairs. The patient himself loses virtually all control over his property and affairs. Guidance must be sought from the Court whenever anything not provided for in an existing order or direction needs to be done (*Re W* 1971). The Court of Protection is not concerned with the patient as a person and therefore it does not deal with matters relating to his care. Of course, the line between matters of welfare and those relating to property may not always be easy to draw in practice, as is demonstrated in divorce cases. Further details relating to the Court of Protection should be sought in the standard textbook (*Heywood and Massey*, 1978 or in *Gostin* 1983).

It should be noted that an incapable patient cannot authorise, by power of attorney or otherwise, any person to act on his behalf. A power of attorney (or agency) is revoked by a patient becoming incapable. But agents and third parties who conclude transactions in ignorance of the revocation may be protected (Powers of Attorney Act 1971, ss.4 and 5).

VIII. *Protection of Patients from Sexual Abuse*

It is an offence for a man of the staff of, or employed by, a hospital or mental nursing home to have extra-marital sexual intercourse with a woman receiving treatment for mental disorder, whether as out- or in-patient, unless he did not know and had no reason to suppose her to be a mentally disordered patient (M.H.A. 1959, s.128). It is also an offence for any man to have extra-marital sexual intercourse with any woman who suffers from severe mental impairment, unless he did not know and had no reason to believe her so to suffer (M.H.A. 1959, s.127). Homosexual acts between males in the same circumstances as those covered by sections 127 and 128 of the 1959 Act are also criminal (Sexual Offences Act 1967, s.1(3) and (4)).

IX. *Removal of Patients from the United Kingdom*

Section 86 of the Mental Health Act 1983, gives the Home Secretary the power to authorise the removal from this country of any patient who is a non-patrial within the meaning of the Immigration Act 1971, who is receiving hospital treatment for mental illness. He must be satisfied that proper arrangements have been made for the care or treatment of the patient in the country to which he is being removed. This is now limited to patients who are detained for treatment or are subject to a hospital order or direction. Further, the Home Secretary has to obtain the approval of a Mental Health Review Tribunal before he can exercise his power to remove a patient in this way (s.86(3)). Any restriction order still in force continues in force so as to apply to the patient if he returns to England and Wales at any time before the end of the period for which the restriction would have continued in force (s.35(3)). There are also provisions for the removal of patients to the Channel Islands and the Isle of Man (M.H.A. 1983, s.83) and for the removal of patients and offenders found insane in the Channel Islands and the Isle of Man to England and Wales (M.H.A. 1983, ss.84, 85).

8. Discharge from Mental Hospitals

A patient who is detained in a mental hospital may be discharged in a number of ways. The Mental Health Act provides for the discharge of detained patients: (i) by the responsible medical officer or hospital managers; (ii) by the nearest relative. A patient may also apply to a Mental Health Review Tribunal (M.H.R.T.). Each of these methods of discharge is considered in turn.

I. Discharge by the Responsible Medical Officer or Hospital Managers

Section 23 of the Mental Health Act 1983 gives responsible medical officers and hospital managers the authority to discharge all detained patients, except mentally disordered offenders with restrictions on their release. In such cases the Home Secretary's consent is required (M.H.A. 1983, s.41(3)(c)(iii)). Such cases apart, the responsible medical officer or hospital managers may discharge a patient at any time. The durations of authority to detain in the Act are statutory maxima. The power to discharge a patient can be exercised at any time prior to the expiration of the maximum period of detention.

The power conferred on the hospital managers may be exercised by any three or more members authorised by them (M.H.A. 1983, s.23(4)). It is rare for hospital managers to make such decisions but their power to do so has not been removed. The responsible medical officer may also grant leave of absence (see below, p.161).

II. *Discharge by the Nearest Relative*

The nearest relative (see above, p.132 for the definition of this) has the power to order the discharge of a patient detained for assessment (above, p.134) or treatment (above, p.136) (M.H.A. 1983, s.25(1)). He is required to give the managers not less than 72 hours notice in writing of his intention to discharge the patient, during which time the responsible medical officer may make a report to the hospital managers certifying that, in his opinion, the patient if discharged "would be likely to act in a manner dangerous to other persons or to himself." This report prevents the relative from discharging the patient for six months (M.H.A. 1983, s.25(1)(*b*)). Where the responsible medical officer furnishes such a report, the nearest relative may, within the following 28 days, apply to a M.H.R.T. requesting the discharge of the patient, (s.66(1)(*g*), (2)(*d*)).

The power of discharge only applies to patients admitted for assessment or treatment under sections 2 or 3 (see M.H.A. 1983, s.23(2)(*a*)), or subject to a guardianship (s.23(2)(*b*)). The nearest relative cannot discharge a patient detained under section 4, nor can he discharge a patient on a hospital order made by a court.

III. *Discharge by Mental Health Review Tribunal*

Proceedings before Mental Health Review Tribunals are governed by the Mental Health Review Tribunal Rules 1983 (S.I. 1983 No. 942). For the details see Chapter 9 (below, p.175). Assistance by way of representation under section 2A of the Legal Aid Act 1974 (see Legal Advice and Assistance (Amendment) Regulations 1982, regs. 3 and 4) has been available since December 1, 1982 to the applicant to the M.H.R.T., whether patient or nearest relative. A "reasonableness" test is being used to determine whether such legal aid should be granted in a particular case. It is too early to assess the impact of this long overdue reform.

The 1982 Act provides (s.41) that patients under the age of 16 can apply to a tribunal.

Eligibility for application to tribunals is dependent on the grounds under which the patient was admitted to hospital.

(a) Admission for assessment

A patient who is admitted to hospital in pursuance of an application for admission for assessment may apply to a M.H.R.T. within 14 days of admission (see M.H.A. 1983, s.66(1)(*a*), (2)(*a*)).

(b) Admission for treatment

(i) A patient who is admitted to hospital for treatment under section 3 may apply to a M.H.R.T. within six months of admission (M.H.A. 1983, s.66(1)(*b*), (2)(*b*)) and thereafter once during each period of detention.

(ii) A patient or nearest relative may apply to a M.H.R.T. within 28 days of receiving notice that the responsible medical officer has reclassified the patient as suffering from a form of mental disorder different from that originally specified in the application (M.H.A. 1983, s.16(1); 66(1)(*d*), (2)(*d*)).

(iii) A nearest relative may apply to a M.H.R.T. within 28 days of receiving notice that a barring certificate (above, p.158) has been made by the responsible medical officer under section 25 of the Mental Health Act 1983 (see s.66(1)(*g*), (2)(*d*)).

(c) Guardianship

Patients under guardianship, and where appropriate their nearest relative, may apply to a M.H.R.T. in the same circumstances as patients under hospital orders or section 3 applications (see (b) above).

(d) Automatic referral

A common criticism in the past has focussed on the small number of those eligible to apply to the tribunals who took advantage of the review procedure. Only 15 per cent. of eligible patients have exercised their rights to appeal to tribunals. It is alleged, with considerable justification, that the law placed too heavy a burden on the patient to take the initiative (*Gostin* 1975, 1980). He was assumed to have "legal competence" (*Carlin* 1966) though often, of course, he was institutionalised, fatalistic and incapable of challenging the system.

The 1982 Act (s.40(1)) accordingly placed a duty on the hospital managers to refer to a tribunal any patient who has been detained for treatment but has not had a tribunal hearing in the first six months of detention, and any patient who has been transferred from guardianship to hospital within six months of his transfer if there has not been a hearing in the interim (see M.H.A. 1983, s.68(1)).

The managers are also required to refer to a M.H.R.T. any patient who has been detained for three years (one year in the case of child patients under 16) without a tribunal hearing (M.H.A. 1983, s.68(2)).

It is also provided that a patient who applies to a M.H.R.T. but withdraws his application "shall be treated as not having exercised his right to apply, and where a person withdraws his application" when six months have elapsed "the managers shall refer his case as soon as possible" to the tribunal (s.68(5)).

The Secretary of State for Social Services also has the power to refer cases to a M.H.R.T. (M.H.A. 1983, s.67(1)). It is a power, and one rarely exercised, and not a duty. The patient whose case is so referred now has the right to call for an independent medical opinion (M.H.A. 1983, s.67(2)).

(e) Powers of a Mental Health Review Tribunal

The tribunal has the power to discharge the patient in any case (M.H.A. 1983, s.72). It must discharge a section 2 patient if it is satisfied that the patient is not then suffering from mental disorder or mental disorder of a nature or degree which warrants his detention in a hospital for assessment (or for assessment followed by medical treatment) for at least a limited period or that his detention as aforesaid is not justified in the interests of his own health or safety or with a view to the protection of other persons (M.H.A. 1983, s.72(1)(*a*)). It must also discharge a patient detained otherwise than under section 2 if satisfied that he is not then suffering from mental illness, psychopathic disorder, mental impairment or severe mental impairment or from any of those forms of disorder of a nature or degree which makes it appropriate for him to be liable to be detained in a hospital for medical treatment or that it is not necessary for the health or safety of the patient or for the protection of other persons that he should receive such treatment, or in the case of an application by the nearest relative of a patient detained under section 3 of the 1983 Act, when the patient's responsible medical officer has issued a report under section 25(1) blocking that relative's discharge powers, that the patient, if released, would not be likely to act in a manner dangerous to other persons or to himself (M.H.A. 1983, s.72(1)(*b*)). A tribunal is not required to discharge a patient detained for treatment even if the "treatability criterion" (or in the case of mental illness or severe mental impairment, the modified "treatability criterion") is not met: the tribunal must only "have regard" to these matters (M.H.A. 1983, s.72(2)).

The 1982 Act extended the range of options open to a tribunal when considering an application. It may direct the discharge of the patient immediately or on a future specified date. Where it does not direct the discharge of a patient, it may, with a view to facilitating his discharge at a future time, recommend (but not, be it noted, "order") that he be granted leave of absence (below, pp. 161–162) or transferred to another hospital or into guardianship. The tribunal may further consider his case in the event of any such recommendation not being complied with (see now M.H.A. 1983, s.72(3)).

Mental Health Review Tribunals also have the power to reclassify the patient, if it is considered that he is suffering from a different form of disorder from that originally specified (M.H.A. 1983, s.72(5). The effect is the same as reclassification by the responsible medical officer under section 16 of the 1983 Act (above, p. 136).

The tribunal's decision must be communicated to the applicant, the patient and the responsible authority within seven days of the hearing (Mental Health Review Tribunal Rules 1983 S.I. 1983 No. 942), r.24(1)). Reasons for the decision must be recorded, and communicated in writing to all the parties. The reasons may be withheld in the patient's interests or for other special reasons (r.24(2)).

IV. *Leave of Absence*

Leave of absence may be granted to any compulsory patient by the responsible medical officer subject to such conditions, if any, as he considers necessary in the interests of the patient or for the protection of other persons (M.H.A. 1983, s.17(1)). For restricted patients the Home Secretary's permission is necessary (M.H.A. 1983, s.41(3)(*c*)). Leave may be granted either indefinitely or on specified occasions (*e.g.* a wedding or funeral), or for any specified period (*e.g.* a weekend). It can be extended by further leave without bringing the patient back to hospital. At any time during an authorised leave of absence, the responsible medical officer may, by written notice given to the patient or to the person temporarily in charge of the patient, recall the patient to the hospital (M.H.A. 1983, s.17(4)). However, where the patient is on an authorised leave of asence for a continuous period of six months, he is no longer subject to recall and he ceases to be liable to be detained (M.H.A. 1983, s.17(5)).

The responsible medical officer, having regard to the interests of the patient or the protection of other persons, may, upon granting leave of absence, direct that the patient "remain in custody during his absence." In which case the patient may be kept in the custody of any officer on the staff of the hospital or of any other person authorised in writing by the hospital managers (M.H.A. 1983, s.17(3)). Where the patient is required, in accordance with conditions imposed on the grant of leave of absence, to reside in another hospital, he may be directed to be kept in the custody of any officer on the staff of that other hospital (M.H.A. 1983, s.17(3)).

V. *Absence without Leave*

A person is absent without leave if he absconds from a hospital to which he has been compulsorily admitted, or fails to return at the expiry of or recall from leave of absence or breaks a residence condition in his leave of absence. He may be taken into custody and returned to the hospital or place (at which he is required to reside) by any approved social worker, any officer on the staff of the hospital, any constable or any person authorised in writing by the hospital managers (M.H.A. 1983, s.18(1)). There is a similar provision regarding guardianship (M.H.A. 1983, s.18(3)). Where a patient is absent without leave from a hospital other than the one in which he is liable to be detained, he can be taken into custody by an officer on the staff of the hospital from which he has absconded or by any person authorised by the managers of that hospital (M.H.A. 1983, s.18(2)).

However, a patient may not be taken into custody and ceases to be liable to detention after a period of 28 days continuous unauthorised absence from the hospital (M.H.A. 1983, s.18(4)). Further, a patient cannot be taken into custody if the period for which he is liable to be detained has expired (M.H.A. 1983, s.18(5)).

It is a criminal offence to induce or knowingly assist a patient to absent himself from hospital without authorisation (M.H.A. 1983, s.128(1)). It is also a criminal offence knowingly to harbour or provide assistance to a patient who is absent without leave (M.H.A. 1983, s.128(3)).

Aftercare

There are two provisions relating to aftercare. The National Health Service Act 1977 states: "A local social services authority may, with the Secretary of State's approval, and to the extent as he may direct shall, make arrangements for the purposes of the prevention of illness and for the care of persons suffering from illness and for the aftercare of persons who have been so suffering" (Sched. 8, para. 2(1)). DHSS Circular No. 19 (para. 4) directs local authorities to provide "centres (including training centres and day centres) or other facilities (including domiciliary facilities), whether in premises managed by the [local authority] or otherwise, for training or occupation of persons suffering from or who have been suffering from mental disorder." The Government thought this provision sufficient and was reluctant to see an aftercare provision included in the 1982 Act. One was, however, added in the House of Lords (it is now M.H.A. 1983, s.117).

This lays a duty on the District Health Authority and the local social services authority, in co-operation with relevant voluntary agencies, to provide aftercare services. The section applies to persons who, having been detained for treatment or under a hospital order or transfer direction, cease to be detained and leave hospital. It does not apply to detained patients granted leave of absence under section 17 of the 1983 Act. "Aftercare" is not defined in the Act. The duty to provide it continues until the District Health Authority and local social services authority are satisfied that the person no longer needs such services (s.117(2)). It is difficult to see how they can be satisfied unless they have closely observed the former patient's progress in the community since his discharge.

A person who alleges that a local social services authority is failing to carry out its duty under section 117 can seek to invoke the Secretary of State's default powers under section 124 of the 1983

Act (see M.H.(A.)A. 1982, s.68(3)(i)). Default powers preclude reliance on any other remedy (*Southwark London Borough Council* v. *Williams* [1971] Ch. 734; *Wyatt* v. *Hillingdon London Borough Council* (1978) 76 L.G.R. 727). It is difficult to see the Secretary of State using his default powers, so that the provision for aftercare in section 117 is little short of unenforceable. (On aftercare generally see *Meacher*, 1979).

9. The Management of Mental Disorder

Approved social workers

One of the most significant changes effected by the 1982 Act (s.61) is the establishment of the concept of approved social workers. As from October 18, 1984 they are to discharge the functions under mental health legislation previously carried out by mental welfare officers. Until that date mental welfare officers will continue to carry out the functions conferred upon them by the 1959 and 1982 Acts (as now consolidated in the 1983 Act).

A local social services authority is to appoint a sufficient number of approved social workers to discharge the functions laid down by the mental health legislation (M.H.A. 1983, s.114). No person is to be appointed as an approved social worker (hereafter A.S.W.) unless he is approved by the authority as having appropriate competence in dealing with persons who are suffering from mental disorder (M.H.A. 1983, s.114(2)). Guidance on what constitutes a "sufficient" number has been given in para. 8 of "Draft Guidelines for Approval of Social Workers Under the Proposed Mental Health (Amendment) Act" published by the DHSS in December 1981: "generally speaking a count of the number of crises referred to the department is likely to be a better indicator than the recorded number of compulsory admissions to hospitals." Although approval is to be undertaken by the social services authorities, training and examination will be superintended by the Central Council for Education and Training in Social Work (C.C.E.T.S.W.). The new legislation thus recognises the key role of the social workers in effecting compulsory admissions to hospital. For the first time since the implementation of the Seebohm

Report (1968) in 1971 the idea of specialist social workers has been statutorily affirmed. The change must be welcomed as a safeguard against the unqualified holding positions of power which have far-reaching consequences for the lives and civil liberties of individual clients, particularly since there is no real judicial surveillance of much mental health decision-making. However, for adequate protection more is required than the good intentions found in the 1982 Amendment Act, as now consolidated: at a time of cutbacks there is a danger that the resources will not be available properly to train enough social workers to carry out the vastly expanded duties envisaged by the new legislation (see also *Meacher*, 1983).

Somewhat ironically, in the light of what has just been said, there is no requirement that the social workers appointed to become A.S.W.s need to be qualified in social work. The Secretary of State has the power to make a direction to this effect under section 114(3) of the 1983 Act. The Government argued that to insert such a requirement would have the effect of excluding a small number of existing mental welfare officers who, while possessing a wealth of relevant experience, have no formal social work qualifications.

It is also rather two-faced to have enhanced the role of social workers while at the same time enabling their skills to be by-passed by retaining the nearest relative's powers to apply for admission to a mental hospital. There are, however, safeguards in such cases (see above, p.133).

Duties and powers of approved social workers

The general duties of the A.S.W. are laid down in section 13 of the 1983 Act. The A.S.W. is placed under a duty to make an application for admission to hospital or a guardianship application, if, having taken into account the wishes expressed by his relatives or any other relevant circumstances, he thinks it necessary or proper for the application to be made by him. As far as patients within the area of the A.S.W.'s authority are concerned, a *duty* is imposed on the A.S.W. but A.S.W.s *may* also make an application in respect of a patient outside his own local social services area (s.13(3)). This additional power caters for the problem that may arise in the evening *or* at weekends if authorities share an out-of-hours service. It also enables an informal patient in a hospital outside the area in which he lives to be detained, should this become necessary.

It should be noted that the duty in section 13(1) is placed on the A.S.W., not the local social services authority. The A.S.W. must exercise independent professional judgment. Obviously, account must be taken of medical opinion but the ultimate decision is the A.S.W.'s. It must be based fairly and squarely on the statutory criteria. Further, the A.S.W. must be able to state the evidence upon which conclusions have been drawn.

Before making an application for the admission of a patient to hospital, the A.S.W. has a duty to interview the patient in a suitable manner and satisfy himself that detention in hospital is, in all circumstances of the case, including past history and present personal, family and social circumstances, the most appropriate way of providing the care and medical treatment which the patient needs. The A.S.W. cannot satisfy himself that detention in hospital is the most appropriate response unless and until alternative arrangements have been explored. This he must do. If detention in hospital is not necessary but alternative community-based resources are not available, the A.S.W. should record this fact on the patient's application.

If an A.S.W. is the applicant in an admission for assessment under section 2 (above, p.134), he must take practicable steps to inform the patient's nearest relative that the application is to be or has been made and of the power of the nearest relative to discharge the patient from hospital under section 23(2)(*a*) (above, p.158) (s.11(3)). In the case of admission for treatment (s.3) or an application for guardianship (s.7), the A.S.W. should consult the nearest relatives before making the application. If the nearest relative objects, the A.S.W. cannot proceed with the application. He can, however, apply to the county court for it to transfer the powers of the nearest relative to another person on the ground (*inter alia*) that the nearest relative "unreasonably objects to the making of an application for admission for treatment or a guardianship application" (s.29(3)(*c*)).

A nearest relative may "require" a local social services authority to consider a patient's case under section 13(1) with a view to making an application for his admission to hospital. It is then the duty of the authority "to direct an approved social worker" as soon as practicable to consider the case. If the A.S.W. decides not to make an application he must inform the nearest relative of his reasons in writing (s.13(4)).

A completed application for the admission of a patient to hospital is sufficient authority for the applicant (or any person authorised by him) to take the patient and convey him to hospital within the time limits provided for by section 6 (as to which see p.132). When carrying out this function the A.S.W. has "all the powers, authorities, protection and privileges" which a constable has in the execution of his duties (s.137(2)) (as to these see *De Smith* 1982). This is enormously wide and will increase when the Police and Criminal Evidence Act 1984 comes into operation (*Freeman* 1984). It must, however, follow from these powers that the A.S.W. also has certain responsibilities akin to those of the police: for example, he must be under a duty to explain the situation to the patient and inform him at least in outline of his rights.

If the patient escapes while being conveyed to hospital the A.S.W. may retake him (s.138).

An A.S.W. may at all reasonable times enter and inspect any premises, except a hospital, in his own local authority area, in which a mentally disordered person is living if he has reasonable cause to believe that the patient is not under proper care. If asked to do so, he must produce his identity card showing him to be an A.S.W. (s.115). The A.S.W. is not entitled under section 115 to force entry if entry is refused. A person who refuses entry to an A.S.W. without reasonable cause commits the offence of obstruction (s.129). If it becomes necessary to force entry, an A.S.W. may apply to a Justice of the Peace for a warrant authorising a constable to enter, if need be by force, any premises specified in the warrant (s.135(1)). The constable must be accompanied by an A.S.W. and a registered medical practitioner (s.135(4)). Similarly, if a patient escapes from an A.S.W.'s custody and is believed to be staying at premises where entry has been denied, the A.S.W. may apply to a J.P. for a warrant under section 135(2). The warrant authorises a constable to enter the premises, if need be by force, and to remove the patient. The constable must be accompanied by a doctor and by any other person authorised to take or retake the patient to hospital (s.135(4)). Such a person could be an A.S.W. but need not be so. Patients removed to a place of safety (as to which see p.131) under section 135 may be detained there for up to 72 hours (s.135(3)).

Approved social workers are also involved when a policeman invokes his power under section 136. This provides that if a constable finds in a public place a person appearing to suffer from a mental disorder who is in immediate need of care or control, he may remove him to a place of safety to protect him or others (see further p.129). The person may then be detained for 72 hours for examination by a registered medical practitioner and for interview by an A.S.W. to make any necessary arrangments for his treatment or care.

An approved social worker has power to take into custody a detained patient who has absented himself from hospital without leave and a patient under guardianship who absents himself without leave of the guardian (s.18). It should be stressed that any A.S.W. has these powers: he does not have to be in the employment of the social services authority responsible for the patient's care. A patient cannot be taken into custody under this provision if he has remained absent without leave for 28 days since the authority to detain him or subject him to guardianship ends at the expiration of that period (s.18(4)).

A further power of A.S.W.s is to make an application to the county court for an order appointing either the local social services authority or a specified individual to act as the patient's nearest relative (s.29(2)(c)). An application can be made on any of the following four grounds:
   (a) the patient has no nearest relative or it is not reasonably practicable to ascertain whether he has or who that relative is;
   (b) the nearest relative is incapable of acting as such by reason of mental disorder or other illness;
   (c) the nearest relative unreasonably objects to the making of an application for treatment or a guardianship application;
   (d) the nearest relative either has or is likely to exercise his power of discharge without due regard to the welfare of the patient or the interests of the public (s.29(3)).
If an order appointing an acting nearest relative has been made, an A.S.W. can apply to the county court for it to be varied (s.30).

A.S.W.s are not involved in the court proceedings that result in a hospital order being made in respect of a mentally disordered offender. However, once such an order is made, an A.S.W. has

the authority to convey the patient to the hospital specified in the
order within a period of 28 days (s.40(1)).

Social reports

Where a patient is admitted to hospital under section 2 (assessment) or section 3 (treatment) following an application by the
nearest relative, the hospital managers must notify the local social
services authority for the area where the patient lived as soon as
practicable and a social worker, who does *not* have to be an
A.S.W. must interview the patient and provide the managers with
a report on the patient's social circumstances (s.14).

Apart from aftercare services (s.117) (see above, p.163) this is
the only function which non-approved social workers may carry
out.

Medical recommendations

Medical recommendations are required to support:
  (i) an application for admission for assessment (s.2(3));
 (ii) an application for admission for treatment (s.3(3));
(iii) emergency applications for admission for assessment
     (s.4(3));
(iv) an application for guardianship (s.7(3)).

In the case of (i), (ii) and (iv) the application must be founded
on the written recommendations of *two* registered medical practitioners. The recommendations may be either separate recommendations, each signed by a registered medical practitioner, or a
joint recommendation signed by two such practitioners (s.11(7)).

In (iii) an application is sufficient in the first instance if founded
on one medical recommendation given, if practicable, by a practitioner who has previous acquaintance with the patient (s.4(3)).
Such emergency applications cease to have effect on the expiration
of a period of 72 hours from the time when the patient is admitted
to hospital unless a second medical recommendation is given and
received by the hospital managers within that period (s.4(4)). Both
recommendations must then comply with the requirements of section 12 (see below), other than the requirement as to the time of
the signature of the second recommendation (s.4(4)(*b*)).

Medical recommendations must:
 (1) be signed on or before the date of application;

(2) be given by practitioners who have personally examined the patient either together or separately (where separately, not more than five days must have elapsed between the days on which the examinations took place, (s.12(1)).

One of the medical recommendations must be given by a practitioner approved by the Secretary of State as having "special experience in the diagnosis or treatment of mental disorder." Unless he also has previous acquaintance with the patient, the other recommendation is, if practicable, to be given by a registered medical practitioner who has (s.12(2)). Where the applicant is a registered medical practitioner he is disqualified from making a medical recommendation (s.12(5)(*a*)): so is a partner of his (s.12(5)(*b*)). Further, the partner of a practitioner who has given a medical recommendation cannot give the second recommendation: nor can a person employed as an assistant by the applicant or by a practitioner who has made the first recommendation. Also disqualified from making a recommendation are persons who receive or have an interest in the receipt of any payments made on account of the maintenance of the patient and practitioners, except part-timers, on the staff of the hospital to which the patient is to be admitted, as well as close family members.

Any application which appears to be duly made and to be founded on the necessary medical recommendations may be acted upon without further proof of the signature or qualification of the person by whom the application or medical recommendation is made or given (s.6(3)). However, if within 14 days of admission for assessment or treatment, it is found that the application is incorrectly completed or if a medical recommendation is incorrect or defective, it may, within that period and with the consent of the hospital's managers, be amended by the person who signed it. Upon such amendment being made the application or recommendation is to have effect (and furthermore shall be deemed to have had effect) as if it had been originally made as so amended (s.15(1)). If it appears to the hospital managers that *one* of the two medical recommendations on which the application is founded is "insufficient to warrant the detention of the patient" they may (that is, there is no mandatory duty on them) give written notice to the applicant. If they do, that recommendation is "disregarded" but the application is to be regarded as "sufficient," if a fresh medical recommendation complying with the Act is furnished to the managers within the period of 14 days beginning with the day on which the patient was admitted and the new recommendation complies with the provisions of the Act (s.15(2)).

Since compliance with time-limits is crucial it may be useful to summarise the procedure once again:

(i) the applicant must have seen the patient within 14 days;

(ii) the dates of the medical examinations must not be more than 5 days apart;

(iii) the dates of the signatures of both medical recommendations must not be later than the date of the application;

(iv) the admission to hospital must take place within 14 days of the date of the later medical recommendation.

Functions of relatives of patients

The terms "relative" and "nearest relative" were explained in an earlier chapter (above, p.132). Various functions are conferred on the patient's relatives in connection with applications for admission and discharge and applications to a M.H.R.T. The nearest relative may authorise some other person to perform his functions (see Mental Health (Hospital, Guardianship and Consent to Treatment) Regulations 1983, reg.14). The selection of the nearest relative is governed by a number of principles:

(i) There is a preference for relatives who ordinarily live with the patient and care for him (see s.26(4)).

(ii) The list of relatives in section 26(1) (see above, p.132) is ranked, so that the nearest relative is the person first described in that list who is surviving (s.26(3)).

(iii) Whole blood relatives are given preference over half blood relatives of the same description (s.26(3)).

(iv) The elder or eldest of two or more relatives is preferred to the other or others of those relatives, regardless of sex (s.26(3)).

(v) A cohabitant of the opposite sex of six months standing is regarded as a spouse (s.26(6)).

(vi) A non-relative who has resided with the patient for five years is treated as a relative but is placed after the relatives listed in section 26(1). He is not given preference over a spouse unless the patient is permanently separated by court order or indefinitely separated by agreement from the spouse (s.26(7)).

There are a number of grounds for by-passing the "nearest relative." They are:

(i) he is not living (is not "ordinarily resident") in the United Kingdom, Channel Islands or Isle of Man;

(ii) he/she is the husband/wife of the patient but is permanently separated (by court order) or indefinitely separated (by agreement) from him/her;

(iii) he/she is under 18, unless he/she is husband, wife, father or mother of the patient;

(iv) an order divesting him of authority over the patient has been made under section 38 of the Sexual Offences Act 1956 and has not been rescinded (s.26(5)).

The nearest relative may make an application for admission for assessment, admission for treatment and a guardianship application. The application must specify the qualification of the applicant to make the application (s.11(1)). The nearest relative must have personally seen the patient within the previous 14 days (s.11(5)), and the hospital managers must seek a social report as soon as practicable (s.14).

The nearest relative may object to an application being made by an A.S.W. To do this he must notify the A.S.W. or the local social services authority by whom that social worker is appointed (s.11(4)). Further, a social worker must not apply, except after consultation with the person, if any, appearing to be the nearest relative of the patient unless it appears to the social worker that in the circumstances such consultation is not reasonably practicable or would involve unreasonable delay (s.11(4)).

The nearest relative also has limited powers to effect the discharge of a patient in cases where the patient is liable to be detained in a hospital in pursuance of an application for admission for assessment, or treatment, or where the patient is subject to guardianship (s.23(2)). There are restrictions on discharge by a nearest relative. He must give 72 hours notice in writing to the hospital managers. If within 72 hours after such notice is given, the responsible medical officer furnishes the hospital managers with a report certifying that in his opinion the patient, if discharged, would be likely to act in a manner dangerous to other persons or to himself, the order for discharge has no effect and no further order for the patient's discharge can be made by the relative during the period of six months commencing with the date of the report (s.25(1)). Where the patient is detained in pursuance of an application for admission for treatment, the hospital managers must see that the nearest relative is informed as to the report (s.25(2)).

The nearest relative also has the power to apply to the M.H.R.T. in the following three cases:

(i) Where a patient is reclassified under section 16. The nearest relative must be informed and he may apply to a M.H.R.T. within 28 days (s.16(4)) (see s.66(1)(*d*), (2)(*d*)).

(ii) Where the responsible medical officer bars discharge by the nearest relative by furnishing a report under section 25 (see above, p.158). The nearest relative must be informed (s.25(2)) and may apply in the 28 days beginning with the day on which he is informed that the report has been furnished (s.66(1)(*g*), (2)(*d*)).

(iii) Where the nearest relative is barred from acting as such by order of the county court under section 29. The relative may apply in the first 12 months of the order and subsequently in each 12 month period for which the order is in force (s.66(1)(*h*), (2)(*g*)).

Hospital managers

If a patient detained in hospital for treatment does not apply to a tribunal and no referral to a tribunal is made on his behalf within the six month period of the compulsory admission or he applies and withdraws his application (as to which see s.68(5)), the hospital managers must then refer his case to a M.H.R.T. (s.68(1)). Subsequently, after any three year period without a tribunal review, or one year if a patient is under 16, the managers must refer the case to a M.H.R.T. (s.68(2)). A doctor authorised by or on behalf of the patient may at any reasonable time visit and examine the patient in private and require the production of and inspect any records relating to the detention or treatment of the patient in hospital (s.68(3)).

The Mental Health Act Commission

The 1982 Act set up as a special health authority a Mental Health Act Commission (see M.H.A. 1983, s.121). The Commission, though having to comply with directions from the Secretary of State, is broadly independent. The selection of its members, however, has proved controversial. Membership includes lawyers, nurses, social workers and psychologists as well as laymen and doctors. The Commission is to be divided into panels in three centres. It is also to have a central policy committee which will be responsible, *inter alia*, for a bi-annual report on the activities of the Commission. This report must be laid by the Secretary of State before Parliament (s.121(10)). The main functions of the M.H.A.C. are:

(i) appointing approved doctors (s.121(2));

(ii) visiting and interviewing patients detained under the Act (s.120(1)); (If a registered medical practitioner, the Commission member may examine the patient. The M.H.A.C. may inspect records relating to detention and treatment of any patient (s.120(4)).)

(iii) investigating complaints by patients or former patients which the Secretary of State considers were not satisfactorily dealt with by the two hospital managers or mental nursing homes (s.120(1));

(iv) investigating complaints by M.P.s (s.120(3));

(v) reviewing the case and treatment of informal patients (s.121(4));

(vi) reviewing decisions to withhold a postal package if

(a) a patient in a special hospital applies to it, complaining that outgoing mail has been stopped under section 134(1)(*b*) (s.121(7)),

(b) a patient or sender of a package applies, complaining that a package has been withheld which was addressed to a patient in a special hospital (as to which see s.134(2)) (s.121(7));

An application in either case must be made within six months of receiving notice that a package is being withheld. The M.H.A.C. may direct that a packet, which is the subject of an application, shall not be withheld. If it does, the hospital managers must comply with the direction (*s*.121(8)).

(vii) reporting to the Secretary of State every second year (and through him to Parliament) (s.121(10)).

The M.H.A.C. has no power to discharge a patient.

Mental Health Review Tribunals

There are M.H.R.T.s in the area of each Regional Health Authority in England and Wales. Each tribunal consists of a legal member, who acts as president, a registered medical practitioner and a person "having such experience in administration, such knowledge of social services or such other qualifications or experience as the Lord Chancellor considers suitable." (M.H.A. 1983, Sched. 2, para. 1(c)). Members of tribunals will be paid remuneration, allowances and expenses.

Sections 66, 69 and 71 of the 1983 Act list the situations where a compulsorily detained patient, and in certain cases his nearest relative, and in others the Secretary of State, may apply to a M.H.R.T. Also listed are the relevant periods within which an application may be made. In each case only one application may be made in the period specified. The main provisions are, in summary form:

Category of Admission	Period of Eligibility
Assessment (s. 66(1)(a))	Within 14 days of admission (patient only)
Treatment (s. 66(1)(b))	Within six months of admission (patient only)
Guardianship (s. 66(1)(c))	Within six months of application being accepted (patient only)
Order barring relative's discharge (s. 25) (s. 66(1)(g))	Within 28 days of being informed (nearest relative only)
Order barring nearest relative from acting as such (s. 29) (s. 66(1)(h))	Within 12 months of order and any subsequent period of 12 months in which order is in force (nearest relative only)
Hospital order (s. 69(1)(a))	After six months (and before 12 months of completion of the order) (by patient or nearest relative). Also in any subsequent period of 12 months.
Guardianship order (s. 69(1)(b))	Within six months by patient. Within 12 months by nearest relative and in any subsequent period of 12 months.
Restricted patient (ss. 70 and 71(1) and (2))	Between six months and 12 months by patient and any subsequent period of 12 months. Any time by Secretary of State. He must if the case has not been heard by a tribunal within the last three years.
Persons detained under Criminal Procedure (Insanity) Act 1964 (s. 71(5))	After six months of order by Secretary of State, if patient himself does not exercise right to apply within six months.

In addition, the Secretary of State for Social Services may at any time refer to a tribunal any patient detained or subject to guardianship under Part II of the 1983 Act (s.67(1)). It cannot be expected that this power will be exercised very often.

Hospital managers have a duty to refer certain cases to a tribunal. If a patient detained in hospital for treatment does not apply to a tribunal and no referral to a tribunal is made on his behalf within the six month period of the compulsory admission, they must refer the case (s.68(1)). Subsequently, after any three year period without a tribunal review (or one year in the cases of patients under 16), they must re-refer the case to a tribunal.

An application to a M.H.R.T. must be made in writing. It must be addressed to the tribunal for the area in which the hospital in which the patient is detained is situated or in which the patient is residing under guardianship, as the case may be (s.77(3)). The application is, whenever possible, to include the following information (see Mental Health Review Tribunal Rules 1983 (S.I. 1983 No. 942), r.3(2)):

(a) the name of the patient;
(b) the patient's address (*e.g.* hospital address, guardian's name and address, etc.);
(c) where the application is made by the nearest relative, the name and address of the applicant and his relationship to the patient;
(d) the section of the Act under which the patient is detained;
(e) the name and address of any representative authorised to act (if none has been authorised, whether the applicant intends to do so or to conduct his own case).

When the tribunal receives the application, it must notify the responsible authority, the patient (if he is not the applicant) and the Secretary of State, if the patient is a restricted patient (S.I. 1983 No. 942, r.4(1)). The responsible authority then has three weeks to send a statement to the tribunal containing the name and age of the patient, his date of admission, his mental disorder, the name of the responsible medical officer and the period which the patient has spent under his care, the dates of previous tribunal hearings, the decisions and reasons, the name and address of the patient's nearest relative, the name and address of any other person who takes a close interest in the patient, details of any leave of absence and other matters that may be of relevant (*e.g.* proceedings in the Court of Protection and any receivership order) (r.6(1)(*a*), Sched. 1, Pt. A). It must also send an up to date medical report, including relevant medical history and a full report on the patient's mental condition (r.6(1)(*b*), Sched. 1, Pt. B), as well as a social circumstances report detailing home and family circumstances, opportunities for employment, housing facilities, availability of community support and medical facilities, and financial position of the patient; and the athority's views on the suitability of the patient for discharge (r.6(1)(*c*), Sched. 1, Pt. B).

Where the patient is a restricted patient the Secretary is required to send the tribunal "a statement of such further information relevant to the application as may be available to him" (r.6(2)).

In the case of conditionally discharged patients, the Secretary of State has six weeks to send a statement (the list of information required is slightly different (see Sched. 1, Pts. C and D).

The responsible authority and Secretary of State may, in their respective statements, place certain information in a separate document, where it is believed that the information should be withheld from the patient on the ground that its disclosure would adversely affect the health or welfare of the patient or others (r.6(4)).

When the tribunal gets the statement, it must send a copy to the patient, or other applicant, excluding any part of the statement which is contained in a separate document (r.6(5)).

Notice of the proceedings must be given to other persons interested, *e.g.* where relevant a guardian, the Court of Protection, etc. (r.7).

Any party may be represented at the hearing by any person whom he has authorised for that purpose "not being a person liable to be detained or subject to guardianship . . . or a person receiving treatment for mental disorder at the same hospital or nursing home as the patient" (r.10(1)). In addition to a representative, a patient or any other party may be "accompanied" by such other person or persons as he wishes (r.10(6)). The tribunal is empowered to authorise a representative for a patient who has omitted to exercise the right to representation (r.10(3)). Legal aid may be available see above, p.158.

The medical member of the tribunal (or at least one of them where there is more than one) must examine the patient before the hearing (r.11).

The tribunal may take evidence on oath and subpoena any witness to appear before it or to produce documents (r.14(1)). It may receive in evidence any document or information notwithstanding that it would be inadmissible in a court of law (r.14(2)).

Fourteen days' notice of the hearing must be given to all parties, and, in the case of a restricted patient, the Secretary of State (para. 20). Proceedings are in private unless the patient requests a public hearing and the tribunal is satisfied that a hearing in public would not be contrary to the interests of the public (r.21(1)). Decisions may be announced immediately and, in any event, must be communicated in writing within seven days of the hearing to all the parties (r.24(1)). However, where the tribunal considers that "full disclosure of the recorded reasons for its decision . . . would adversely affect the health or welfare of the patient or others" it may instead communicate the decision in such manner as it considers appropriate (r.24(2)).

On the powers of tribunals to direct the discharge of patients see above, p.158.

10. The Mentally Disordered Offender

Introduction

In this chapter, we consider the admission to mental hospital of mentally disordered offenders and their discharge therefrom. The law relating to such offenders has been the subject of much criticism, notably in the Butler Committee Report on *Mentally Abnormal Offenders* (Cmnd. 6244, 1975) and in the second volume of the Mind publication, *A Human Condition* (*Gostin*, 1977). The law has been recently reformed to take account of these criticisms and to implement some of the recommendations made in the Butler Report and by Gostin. One of the most significant changes has resulted from the decision of the European Court of Human Rights in the case of *X* v. *United Kingdom* (1982) 7 E.L. Rev. 435.

This chapter does not deal with police powers (which are considered above). Nor are matters relating to the trial of mentally disordered offenders considered. For these the reader is referred elsewhere (*Hoggett*, 1984).

(a) Hospital orders

Until 1959, the power to send mentally disordered offenders to hospital applied only to mental defectives. The Mental Health Act 1959 extended this power to a wide range of mentally disordered offenders. A number of changes were effected by the 1982 Amendment Act.

For a hospital order to be made by a Crown Court, the person must have been convicted of an offence punishable with imprisonment other than one for which the sentence is fixed by law (M.H.A. 1983, s.37(1)). In practice this excludes the making of hospital orders on convicted murderers. The Crown Court must actually convict the offender, unless he has been transferred from prison to hospital before trial (M.H.A. 1983, ss.48 and 50). A magistrates' court may make a hospital order without recording a conviction, where the person suffers from mental illness or severe mental impairment, if satisfied that he committed the act or omission with which he has been charged (M.H.A. 1983, s.37(3)). This provides magistrates with a functional equivalent to finding the defendant unfit to plead or not guilty by reason of insanity, neither of which verdicts is open to magistrates' courts.

The court (whether Crown or magistrates') must be satisfied, on the written or oral evidence of two medical practitioners, that the offender is suffering from mental illness, psychopathic disorder, mental impairment or severe mental impairment and that the disorder is of "a nature or degree which makes it appropriate for him to be detained in a hospital for medical treatment and, in the case of psychopathic disorder or mental impairment, that such treatment is likely to alleviate or prevent a deterioration in his condition" (M.H.A. 1983, s.37(2)(a)(i)). The court must also be of the opinion that, considering all the circumstances, including the nature of the offence and the character and antecedents of the offender and other available methods of disposal, a hospital order is the most suitable method of disposal (s.37(2)(b)). Further, the court must be satisfied, on the written or oral evidence of the medical practitioner who would be in charge of the treatment of the patient or some other person representing the hospital managers (who need not be medically qualified), that arrangements have been made for the admission of the offender to a specified hospital within a period of 28 days from the making of the order (M.H.A. 1983, s.37(4)). One of the two medical practitioners giving evidence must be approved under M.H.A. 1983, s.12(2) as having special experience in the diagnosis or treatment of mental disorder (M.H.A. 1983, s.54(1)). The two doctors giving evidence may be from the same hospital (*cf.* the position as regards civil admissions above). A written report by a doctor or a representative of the hospital managers may be admitted as evidence without proof of the signature or proof that he is qualified to give evidence. The signatory may, however, be required to give oral evidence by the court (s.54(2)). Copies of reports must be given to the defendant's representative, if he has one. If he is not represented, the substance of the report must be disclosed to him or, where he is a child or young person, conveyed to his parent or guardian if present in court. Except where the report relates only to arrangements for his admission to hospital, the subject of the report may require its signatory to be called to give oral evidence and evidence to rebut the evidence contained in the report may be called by or on behalf of him (M.H.A. 1983, s.54(3)(c)).

Where the court is minded to make a hospital order or interim hospital order, it may request a Regional Health Authority (or the Secretary of State in Wales) to furnish it with information with respect to the hospitals in its region or elsewhere at which arrangements could be made for the person's admission (M.H.A. 1983, s.39). This provision is a response to concern about difficulties which sometimes arise in finding hospital places for mentally disordered people who appear before the courts.

The effect of a hospital order is very similar to a section 3 admission for treatment (above). It places the person in hospital for a period of up to six months, which can be renewed for another six months and for periods of one year at a time. Provisions relating to reclassification, leave of absence, absconders and discharge by the hospital or responsible medical officer apply (see above). There are, however, some pertinent differences. If the patient is under a hospital order, the nearest relative has no power to discharge him. The nearest relative has, however, the right to apply to a M.H.R.T. "in the period between the expiration of six months and the expiration of 12 months beginning with the date of the order and in any subsequent period of 12 months" (M.H.A. 1983, s.69(1)(a)). Also, the patient is not eligible to apply to a tribunal within the first six months of admission. His periods of eligibility are the same as those which apply to his "nearest relative." Hospital order patients formerly had the right to apply to a tribunal in the first six months but this right was removed by the 1982 Act, as a result of, what appears to be, a strained interpretation of the European Court of Human Rights decision in *X* v. *United Kingdom* (1982). The Government reasoned that hospital order patients will usually have had the appropriateness of their admission and detention tested in the near past by a court. This is not a convicing explanation for depriving patients of an additional power of review (see also *Gostin, The Times*, 1982). Some hospital order patients have not recently received a court review (restricted patients whose restrictions expire or are removed; patients transferred from prison to hospital subject to restrictions (M.H.A. 1983, ss.46(3), 48(3), or 52(3)); those whose restrictions subsequently expire (M.H.A. 1983, s.41(5)); patients transferred to the English hospital system from Scotland, Northern Ireland, the Isle of Man or the Channel Islands (M.H.A. 1983, ss.82(2), 84(2), 85(2)). They are entitled to apply to a M.H.R.T. within the first six months commencing with the date of the hospital order (M.H.A. 1983, s.69(2)). The reasons for this were given by Lord Belstead in the House of Lords debate (Hansard H.L., Vol. 427, col. 868).

(b) Restriction orders

Restriction orders can only be made by a Crown Court. A magistrates' court which believes that restrictions should be imposed can commit an offender over the age of 14 years who has been convicted of an offence punishable on summary conviction with imprisonment to the Crown Court with a view to this being done (M.H.A. 1983, s.43(1)). If the magistrates' court is satisfied, on written or oral evidence, that arrangements have been made for the admission of the offender to a hospital, in the event of an order being made, it may direct him to be admitted to that hospital until the case is disposed of by the Crown Court (M.H.A. 1983, s.44(1)). The alternative is to commit him in custody. About a quarter of hospital orders contain restrictions.

The Crown Court may make a restriction order when it makes a hospital order and considers, having regard to the nature of the offence, the antecedents of the offender and the risk of his committing further offences if set at large, that it is necessary for "the protection of the public from serious harm" so to do (M.H.A. 1983, s.41(1)). Restriction orders (the term itself originates in the 1982 Act) are a compromise between exclusive reliance on therapeutic considerations and the public interest in protection. The Court of Appeal has stressed that courts should have compelling reasons if they do not impose restrictions in the cases of crimes of violence or more serious sexual offences, particularly if the offender has a record of such offences or a history of mental disorder involving violent behaviour (*R. v. Gardiner*, 1967).

The restriction order may either be without limit of time or for a specified period. If it is for a fixed term, the patient is detained under a hospital order without restrictions when the term expires or otherwise ceases to have effect. In *R*. v. *Gardiner* (1967) the court directed that restriction orders of fixed duration should only be made in exceptional cases where doctors are able to assert confidently that recovery will take place within a certain period. This is supported by the Butler Committee. Most restriction orders are accordingly made for unlimited periods.

The Home Secretary can direct that restrictions be lifted at any time, if he is satisfied that they are no longer necessary for the protection of the public from serious harm (M.H.A. 1983, s.42(1)). If restrictions are removed, the order becomes an ordinary hospital order. The Home Secretary may also discharge a restricted patient subject to conditions (s.42(2)). Where he does this he may, at any time during the continuance of the order, recall the patient by warrant to hospital (s.42(3)). The effect of this will be to detain the patient as if the original restriction order were still operative. The European Commission of Human Rights found this procedure to be in breach of Article 5(2) of the European Convention (a person must be informed promptly of the reasons for his arrest). The Government's response has been to issue circulars to the police, probation service and hospitals introducing a two-stage procedure for informing patients of their recall to hospital.

Until the passing of the 1982 Act a person detained under a restriction order had no right to appeal to a M.H.R.T. The law was changed by the 1982 Act to give effect to a decision of the European Court of Human Rights in *X* v. *United Kingdom*. This held that the then exclusive powers of the Home Secretary to discharge a restricted patient were in breach of Article 5(4) of the Convention which requires that a person detained by reason of "unsoundness of mind" must have the opportunity of periodic judicial review of the substantive justification of his detention. As a result of this, it is provided in section 70 of the 1983 Act that a restricted patient may apply to a M.H.R.T. in the period between the expiration of six months and the expiration of 12 months beginning with the date of the relevant hospital order or transfer direction and in any subsequent period of 12 months.

Tribunals have the power to order the absolute or conditional discharge of a restricted patient. The Government has said that when a tribunal is considering the case of a restricted patient it should be chaired by a lawyer with substantial judicial experience in the criminal courts (Hansard H.L., Vol. 426, col. 761). This would normally be a circuit judge, but could also be a recorder.

A M.H.R.T. must direct the *absolute* discharge of the patient if satisfied that: (a) he is not suffering from one of the four forms of mental disorder of a nature or degree which makes it appropriate for him to be liable to be detained in hospital for medical treatment *or* that it is not necessary for the health or safety of the patient *or* for the protection of other persons that he should receive such treatment; *and* (b) that it is not appropriate for him to remain liable to be recalled to hospital for further treatment (M.H.A. 1983, s.73(1)). If the tribunal is satisfied that (a) is met, but not (b), it must direct the *conditional* discharge of the patient (M.H.A. 1983, s.73(2) of the 1983 Act). A patient who is conditionally discharged must comply with any conditions imposed upon him at the time of his discharge or at any subsequent time by the Home Secretary (M.H.A. 1983, s.73(4)(*b*)). A tribunal may defer a direction for the conditional discharge of a patient until such arrangements as appear to the tribunal to be necessary for that purpose have been made to its satisfaction (M.H.A. 1983, s.73(7)). Where by virtue of any such deferment no direction has been given, on an application or reference before the tribunal on a subsequent application or reference, the previous application or reference shall be treated as one on which no direction can be given. Where a patient is *absolutely* discharged by a M.H.R.T., both the hospital order and restriction order cease to have effect (s.73(3)). Where he is *conditionally* discharged, he may be recalled to hospital by the Home Secretary (s.73(4)(*a*)).

Restricted patients have one further protection. The responsible medical officer is required to examine and report to the Home Secretary on such patients at intervals not exceeding one year. Every report is to contain such particulars as the Home Secretary requires (M.H.A. 1983, s.41(6)).

(c) The transfer of prisoners to hospital

The Home Secretary is authorised to transfer a person serving a sentence of imprisonment to a hospital (M.H.A. 1983, s.47), but not a mental nursing home. He must be satisfied by reports of at least two registered medical practitioners, one of whom is "approved" under section 12 (see M.H.A. 1983, s.54(1)), that the prisoner is suffering from one of the four specific forms of mental disorder, *and* that the disorder is of a nature or degree which makes it appropriate for him to be detained in hospital for medical treatment. In the case of the minor disorders (above), the treatment must be likely to alleviate or prevent a deterioration of the condition. The Home Secretary must also consider that it is expedient to make a transfer direction, having regard to the public interest and all the circumstances.

A transfer direction has the same effect as a restriction order (M.H.A. 1983, s.47(3)). Such a direction may be made with or without restrictions on discharge (M.H.A. 1983, s.49(1)). In most cases restrictions on discharge are imposed. A transfer is more likely to be made without restrictions if the prisoner is nearing the end of his sentence. Where the Home Secretary is notified by the responsible medical officer, any other medical practitioner or a M.H.R.T. that the offender no longer requires treatment in hospital for mental disorder or that no effective treatment for his disorder can be given in the hospital to which he has been removed, he can discharge him if he would have been eligible for release on parole or he can direct that he be remitted to prison to serve the rest of his sentence (M.H.A. 1983, s.50(1)). The restriction direction ceases to have effect if the offender is still in hospital on the date on which he could have been discharged if he had not forfeited remission of any part of the sentence after his removal to hospital (M.H.A. 1983, s.50(2), (3)).

Persons detained in a prison or remand centre who are not serving a sentence of imprisonment can also be transferred to hospital by the Home Secretary (M.H.A. 1983, s.48(2)). Three types of prisoner must be considered: (i) civil prisoners; (ii) persons detained under the Immigration Act 1971; and (iii) unsentenced and untried defendants.

In all these cases, the Home Secretary must be satisfied by reports of two medical practitioners, one of whom must be "approved" under section 12 of the 1983 Act, that the prisoner is suffering from mental illness or severe mental impairment of "a nature or degree which makes it appropriate for him to be detained in a hospital for medical treatment" and that he is in "urgent need" of such treatment (M.H.A. 1983, s.48(1)). A person who is the subject of a transfer direction under section 48 must be admitted to the hospital specified in the direction within 14 days (s.47(2), 48(3)).

A transfer direction has the same effect as a hospital order. The Home Secretary must make a restriction direction, save in cases of civil prisoners or persons detained under the Immigration Act 1971, where he may do so.

In the case of an unsentenced or untried defendant whose case has not been disposed of by the Crown Court, a transfer direction ceases to have effect when the case is disposed of by the court. At any time before the case is disposed of, the responsible medical officer, any other medical practitioner or the M.H.R.T. may notify the Home Secretary that the defendant no longer requires treatment in hospital for mental disorder or that no effective treatment can be given. The Home Secretary may respond to this by remitting the defendant to any place where he might have been detained (s.51(3)). If he does this, the transfer direction ceases to have effect. If he does not place the defendant back in custody, the court itself may do so, or may release him on bail, if it is satisfied, on the evidence of the responsible medcial officer, that the person concerned no longer requires treatment in hospital for mental disorder or that no effective treatment can be given. If the court does either remand in custody or release on bail, the transfer direction ceases to have effect (s.51(4)).

In the case of civil prisoners and persons detained under the Immigration Act 1971, the transfer direction ceases to have effect on the expiration of the period during which he would be liable to be detained in the place from which he was removed (M.H.A. 1983, s.53(1)). Where both a transfer direction and a restriction direction have been given, and the Home Secretary is notified by the responsible medical officer, any other medical practitioner or a M.H.R.T. that the person no longer requires treatment in hospital for mental disorder or that no effective treatment for his disorder can be given, he may direct that he be remitted to any place where he might have been detained. The restriction direction ceases on that person's arrival at that place (M.H.A. 1983, s.53(2)).

Persons remanded to custody by a magistrates' court may also be transferred to hospital. In such cases the transfer direction ceases to have effect at the expiration of the period of remand, unless the defendant is committed in custody to the Crown Court (M.H.A. 1983, s.52(2)). A magistrates' court may further remand an accused person (Magistrates' Courts Act 1980, s.129) but not in his absence unless he has appeared before the court within the previous six months. Where a magistrates' court is satisfied, on the evidence of the responsible medical officer, that the defendant no longer requires treatment in hospital for mental disorder or that no effective treatment can be given, it may direct that the transfer direction shall cease to have effect (M.H.A. 1983, s.52(5)).

(d) Remand to hospital for report

Both the Crown Court and magistrates' court have the power to remand an accused person to hospital for a report on his mental condition if satisfied, on the evidence, written or oral, of an approved medical practitioner that: (i) there is reason to suspect that he is suffering from one of the four forms of mental disorder, and (ii) it would be impracticable for a report on his mental condition to be made if he were remanded on bail (M.H.A. 1983, s.35(3)). Courts cannot remand to hospital unless satisfied, on the written or oral evidence of the medical practitioner who would be responsible for making the report or of some other person representing the hospital managers, that arrangements have been made for his admission to hospital within a period of seven days after the remand. If the court is so satisfied it may, pending his admission, give directions for his conveyance to, and detention in, a place of safety (for the meaning of which see above) (M.H.A. 1983, s.35(4)). Courts may further remand an accused person, where this is necessary for completing an assessment of his mental condition, and may do so without his being brought before the court, so long as he is legally represented and his solicitor or counsel is given an opportunity of being heard (M.H.A. 1983, s.35(5), (6)). A remand or a further remand may not be for more than 28 days at a time or for more than 12 weeks in all. The court may at any time terminate the remand if it appears to the court that it is appropriate to do so (M.H.A. 1983, s.35(7)). A person remanded for report is entitled to obtain, at his own expense, an independent report on his mental condition from a medical practitioner chosen by him and to apply to the court on the basis of it for his remand to be terminated (M.H.A. 1983, s.35(8)). This is unlikely to be of much benefit to the accused person. It is doubtful whether the court will be prepared to end remands on the basis of such independent reports.

A person who absconds from a hospital to which he has been remanded under section 35, or while being conveyed to or from that hospital, may be arrested without warrant. He must then be brought before the court that remanded him, as soon as this is practicable. The court may thereupon terminate the remand and may remand him to prison (M.H.A. 1983, s.35(10)).

A person remanded to hospital for a report on his mental condition retains his common law rights to refuse treatment. This is because the consent to the treatment provisions in the 1983 Act do not apply to patients liable to be detained by virtue of section 35 (see M.H.A. 1983, s.56(1)(*b*)).

(e) Remand to hospital for treatment

A Crown Court may, instead of remanding an accused person in custody, remand him to hospital, if satisfied, on the written or oral evidence of two medical practitioners (one of whom is "approved" under M.H.A. 1983, s.12), that he is suffering from mental illness or severe mental impairment of a nature or degree which makes it appropriate for him to be detained in a hospital for medical treatment (M.H.A. 1983, s.36(1)). This power does not apply to persons accused of murder (M.H.A. 1983, s.36(2)). The court must first be satisfied that arrangements have been made for admission to hospital (s.36(3)). There are powers for further remands even in the absence of the accused person, so long as he is legally represented (M.H.A. 1983, s.36(5)). The total duration of remands is as for remands to hospital for reports (above, p.188) (M.H.A. 1983, s.36(6)). The accused person may obtain at his own expense an independent report on his mental condition and may apply on the basis of it for his remand to be terminated (M.H.A. 1983, s.36(7)). The law relating to absconding is similar to that on remands to hospital for reports.

A person remanded for treatment is subject to the provisions on consent to treatment set out in Part IV of the 1983 Act (on which see above).

(f) Interim hospital orders

Where a person is convicted before the Crown Court of an offence punishable with imprisonment, other than murder, or by a magistrates' court of an offence punishable on summary conviction with imprisonment, and the court before or by which he is convicted is satisfied, on the written or oral evidence of two medical practitioners (one of whom is "approved" under the M.H.A. 1983, s.12) that (i) he is suffering from one of the four forms of mental disorder; and (ii) there is reason to suppose that the mental disorder from which he is suffering is such that it may be appropriate for a hospital order to be made, the court may make an interim hospital order. This authorises the offender's admission to hospital and his detention there. (M.H.A. 1983, s.38(1)). Such an order may only be made where the court is satisfied, on the evidence of the medical practitioner who would be in charge of the treatment or another representative of the hospital managers, that arrangements have been made for the offender's admission to hospital within 28 days. If the court is so satisfied it may, pending the admission, give directions for the offender's conveyance to, and detention in, a place of safety (M.H.A. 1983, s.38(4)). An interim hospital order remains in force, for a period not exceeding 12 weeks, which the court specifies. It may be renewed by the court for further periods of 28 days after hearing evidence from the responsible medical officer. It cannot, however, remain in force for more than six months in all. It is to terminate if the court makes a hospital order or decides to deal with the offender in some other way (M.H.A. 1983, s.38(5)). The power of renewing an interim hospital order may be exercised without the offender being brought before the court, so long as he is legally represented and his solicitor or counsel is given an opportunity of being heard (M.H.A. 1983, s.38(6)). The law relating to absconding is as for remands to hospital for reports or treatment.

A person given an interim hospital order is subject to the consent to treatment provisions in Part IV of the 1983 Act (on which see above).

(g) Mental condition of persons accused of murder

A person accused of murder is rarely granted bail. Where he is, it is now provided (by M.H.(A.)A. 1982, s.34, amending the Bail Act 1976) that the court must impose a requirement that: (i) he undergo examination by two medical practitioners for the purpose of enabling reports on his mental condition to be made; (ii) he attend an institution or place as directed by the court to enable the reports to be prepared. At least one of the medical practitioners must be "approved" under section 12 of the 1983 Act. This new provision should assist the proper investigation of possible defences, particularly diminished responsibility (Homicide Act 1957, s.2). On the sentencing process and mentally disordered offenders generally see Ashworth and Gostin (1984).

Part III
The Elderly, the Sick and the Handicapped

11. Residential Accommodation for the Elderly and Physically Handicapped

This is not the place to consider what good social work practice towards the elderly and physically handicapped should be. Suffice it to say that social workers are in the main providing the elderly in particular with basic practical services. Goldberg *et al.* (1977) found in a study of an area office in Southampton that 84 per cent. of elderly and physically disabled clients referred received some form of practical help. The evidence also suggests a higher level of satisfaction with the assistance given amongst the elderly than in the case of younger clients. One of the main factors governing demand for assistance from social services by the elderly is the availability, or absence, of support from family or friends. If the old need help they are more likely to obtain it from a spouse, a child or some other relative, than from social services. Age Concern (1974) found that in personal care tasks, relatives were nearly always more important than health or social workers and, further, the elderly preferred to take their worries to relatives. Some nevertheless do resort to social services and do need the assistance that social workers can provide or provide the key to.

The majority of the elderly are able to continue to live an integrated life in their own home and community. Residential care is an appropriate answer to the needs of a minority. As with children institutional care is no panacea. It may remove the elderly from some hazards only to subject them to others. The elderly must be free to choose whether they remain in their own homes, with relatives or come into residential accommodation but this freedom must be balanced with the freedom of others and related to the risks involved in alternative environments. Since residential accommodation is limited local authorities operate priority grading systems based on the risk concept. Careful planning is desirable but difficult to operationalise when so many cases present themselves as emergencies (*DHSS*, 1976). In the case of non-emergencies doubt has often been expressed (*e.g.* by Brocklehurst *et al*, 1978) as to whether it was necessary to admit the elderly person concerned to residential care. As Brearley notes (1980): "It does seem likely that some people enter care without there being a full consideration of the options."

I. *Purpose of Residential Accommodation for Elderly People*

The Department of Health and Social Security defines the function of a home for elderly people as being:

> "to provide considerate and skilful care in comfortable surroundings for elderly people who, even with help, are unable to live in homes of their own. The primary aim is accordingly to create an atmosphere in which residents can, as an alternative to their own homes live as normally as possible and in which their individuality, independence and personal dignity are respected." (*DHSS Local Authority Building* Note No. 2, May 1973).

Other related functions of a home for the elderly identified by the DHSS include: (a) forming a part of the community from which residents come and to maintain links with local communities; (b) planning for changes in the characteristics of those needing help over a given period enabling residents to use their facilities as fully as they wish to and can; (c) where appropriate, provide a temporary period of residence for an elderly person who needs rest and recuperation or whose relatives need a respite from care or an opportunity for a holiday.

The above functions do not in themselves constitute legal requirements placed upon local authorities, but are guidelines provided by the DHSS for the planning and building of residential accommodation for elderly people. A memorandum on the Care of the Elderly in Hospitals and Residential Homes, issued by the Ministry of Health in 1965 (Circular 10/65) states that the objects of a local authority in providing residential services should be:

"(i) to provide, whether directly or by arrangement with a voluntary body or other local authority, residential accommodation on a scale recorded as adequate to meet the needs as they arise, jointly assessed from time to time with the other branches of the health service. This should be in homes normally of thirty to fifty places sited wherever possible so that close links with the resident's home community are maintained, and designed to provide an informal environment for people who can suitably live together, along with all necessary services;

(ii) while endeavouring as far as is reasonable and practicable to accommodate in these homes people with physical handicaps, difficult personalities or confusion of mind, to provide separate small homes, normally of not more than thirty-five places for people with special needs, including elderly mentally infirm people who are found to be so disturbed that they cannot suitably live with other residents."

To achieve these objects, the Ministry of Health Circular goes on to suggest that local authorities should aim:

"(a) to bring together the available information about elderly people in their area who may come to need residential care; (b) to maintain the independence of the elderly person in the community including special housing for as long as possible, and to plan on the available information for those who are unable to maintain an independent life style; (c) to secure a close association between the homes and the Community Physician in the area; (d) to ensure that the staffing of each home is sufficient to provide proper care for each resident, and that as full a range of health and welfare services is available as if they were in their own homes; (e) to regard 'care and attention' as a positive and not as a residual function."

Each resident should have a personal doctor, and there should be good arrangements for summoning medical and nursing aid if need be.

II. *Categories of Resident*

The category of resident that local authorities may need to admit to homes for the elderly was broadly defined by the 1965 Circular as being "those who are found after careful assessment of their medical and social needs, to be unable to maintain themselves in their own homes, even with full support from outside, but who do not need continuous care by nursing staff." This broad definition is so framed as to include people so incapacitated that they need help with dressing, toilet and meals but who are able to get about with a walking aid or with some help by wheelchair; people using appliances that they can manage themselves or without nursing assistance; as well as people with temporary or continuing confusion of mind but who do not need psychiatric nursing care.

III. *Provision of Residential Accommodation*

The provision of residential accommodation for the elderly and physically handicapped is provided for in Part III of the National Assistance Act 1948. For this reason, such accommodation is often referred to as "Part III Accommodation."

It is the duty of every local authority to provide residential accommodation for persons who "by reason of age, infirmity or any other circumstances are in need of care and attention which is not otherwise available to them" (National Assistance Act 1948, s.21(1)(*a*)). It is the duty of local authorities to have regard to the welfare of all persons for whom accommodation is provided and to provide different kinds of accommodation appropriate to different categories of need (N.A.A. 1948, s.21(2)). Provision may also be made for conveying persons to and from the accommodation provided and for the provision of some health services within the home (N.A.A. 1948, s.21(7)).

Residential accommodation for elderly and physically handicapped persons is not provided free of charge and local authorities may fix a standard rate for the accommodation they provide. However, where a resident satisfies the authority that he is unable to pay the standard fixed rate, the authority is under a duty to assess his ability to pay and to agree to payment at a specified lower rate

(N.A.A. 1948, s.22). The minimum charge is currently fixed at £26.30 per week (S.I. 1982 No. 1399). This means that residents in a local authority home or hostel may be paying at different rates for the same accommodation and services. This may, understandably, lead to some friction between residents, particularly if some feel they are being penalised for their efforts and/or thrift in the past. But there is no other politically acceptable solution.

In assessing a person's ability to pay, a local authority is to take account of that person's needs for personal requirements and to discount "such sum per week as may be prescribed by the Minister" for pocket money (N.A.A. 1948, s.22(4)). The sum currently prescribed is £6.55 per week (S.I. 1982 No. 1399). Where residents receive state pensions or supplementary benefits, payment may be made direct to the local authority by the DHSS in cases where the resident has failed to pay any sum due from him in respect of accommodation provided.

The Health and Social Services and Social Security Adjudications Act 1983 provides (in s.20(1)) that if a local authority thinks fit it has the power to limit to the minimum weekly prescribed rate the payments required for accommodation irrespective of the means of the person concerned. But the authority may only exercise this power for a maximum period of eight weeks commencing when accommodation is provided. The power can nevertheless be exercised on each occasion when accommodation is provided for a person.

The 1983 Act also strengthens the hands of local authorities in their efforts to recover payments from defaulting residents. First, it provides that where a person avails himself of Part III accommodation and "knowingly and with the intention of avoiding charges" has transferred cash or any other asset to some other person or persons not more than six months before the date on which he takes up residential accommodation or transfers any such asset while residing in the accommodation for no consideration or no true consideration, "the person or persons to whom the asset is transferred by the person availing himself of the accommodation shall be liable to pay to the local authority . . . the difference between the amount assessed as due to be paid for the accommodation . . . and the amount which the local authority receive from him for it" (s.21(1)).

Secondly, the 1983 Act provides that where a person who avails himself of Part III accommodation fails to pay any sum assessed for the accommodation and has a beneficial interest in land in England or Wales, the local authority may create a charge in its favour on the interest in the land (s.22(1)). The charge is created by a declaration in writing made by the local authority (s.22(7)). In the case of unregistered land, a Class B land charge within the meaning of section 2 of the Land Charges Act 1972 is created: in the case of registered land a registrable charge taking effect as a charge by way of legal mortgage (s.22(8)). There is a parallel provision dealing with land in Scotland (s.23).

The local authority may make rules as to the conduct of premises under its management and as to the preservation of order in the premises (N.A.A. 1948, s.23(1)). These rules may apply to the circumstances in which people may be required to leave the accommodation or the waiving of part of the payments due for residents who assist in the running of the premises (N.A.A. 1948, s.23(2) and (3)). As far as rules as to the conduct of premises are concerned, local authorites are required (by the N.A.A. 1948, s.35(2)) to exercise their functions under the general guidance of the Secretary of State for Social Services. Guidance has been given by means of Circulars (for example, Circulars 87/48 and 150/48).

The Supplementary Benefits Commission has the power (under the N.A.A. 1948, s.25) to require a local authority to provide accommodation in urgent cases (N.A.A. 1948, s.25). An aggrieved local authority may appeal to the Supplementary Benefits Appeal Tribunal. Where accommodation is provided in this way, the person so accommodated cannot be required to leave the premises except with the consent of the S.B.C. or, where it refuses to give its consent, with the consent of the Supplementary Benefits Appeal Tribunal (N.A.A. 1948, s.25(2)).

A local authority may exercise its duty to provide accommodation by making arrangements with a voluntary organisation to manage any premises for the provision of accommodation. The voluntary organisation is paid by the local authority in respect of the accommodation provided. The local authority may make contributions to the funds of the voluntary organisation which provides accommodation for this purpose. Where this arrangement operates, the local authority may authorise a person or persons to enter and inspect the premises at any reasonable time (N.A.A. 1948, s.26).

IV. *Persons in Need of Care and Attention*

Most elderly persons who enter residential care do so voluntarily, at least that is without any legal procedures being invoked to secure their admission. There is, however, one procedure by which elderly people can be compelled to enter a residential establishment. This procedure (in N.A.A. 1948, s.47, as amended by the National Assistance (Amendment) Act 1951) applies not only to the elderly but also to persons suffering from a grave chronic disease or being physically incapacitated, provided in any case that person is also not receiving proper care and attention, and is living in insanitary conditions.

The origins of the provision are in the Poor Law and are tied up with public health measures. In particular the legislation can be traced to social measures to facilitate slum clearance (*Grey*, 1979). The reference in the contemporary legislation to insanitary conditions is clearly a legacy of this.

The legislation (N.A.A. 1948, s.47) provides that where a person is suffering from a grave chronic disease, or is aged, infirm or physically incapacitated *and* is living in insanitary conditions *and* is not receiving proper care and attention, the local authority may, on receiving medical confirmation, apply to the local magistrates' court or authorise the community physician to do so. The action will have been initiated by the community physician. He must undertake a thorough inquiry and consideration of the person's situation and decide whether it is necessary to remove him either in his own interests or to prevent injury to the health of, or serious nuisance to, other persons. He may then certify his findings in writing and must, if possible, obtain the consent of a manager of suitable premises to take the person in. It is this report which forms the basis of the application to the magistrates' court for an order to be made removing the person to a suitable hospital or other place for a period not exceeding three months (this period may be extended by the court from time to time, on each occasion for a maximum period of three months, in effect indefinitely). The person to be removed, or the person in charge of him, must be given seven clear days notice of the application.

In some circumstances it is possible to remove a person without giving him notice. If the community physician and another doctor consider that it is necessary in the interests of the person concerned to remove him without delay, an application can be made either to the local magistrates' court or to a single justice under section 1(3) of the National Assistance (Amendment) Act 1951 to have him removed. An order may then be made in the absence of the person concerned, in the absence even of any legal representation.

There are no national statistics published on the use of s.47 or s.1(3). It is suspected that there will be wide regional variations since so much will be on the way different community physicians interpret their powers and also, probably, upon local resources. Surprisingly little concern has been expressed as to the operation of these coercive powers. There is clear potential for injustice and infringement of civil liberties.

V. *Protection of Property*

Where a person is admitted as a patient to any hospital, any Part III accommodation, or is removed to any other place under section 47 of the 1948 Act, the local authority has a duty to take reasonable steps to prevent or mitigate the loss of, or damage to, any movable property which the individual is no longer able to protect. For this purpose, the local authority has the power to enter, at all reasonable times, the premises which were the place of residence of the person in hospital or other accommodation (N.A.A. 1948, s.48).

VI. *Welfare Services*

A number of additional powers exist which enable local authorities to promote the welfare of the disabled and elderly.

Local authorities have the power to make arrangements for promoting the welfare of the blind, deaf or dumb and other persons "who are substantially and permanently handicapped by illness, injury or congenital deformity or such other disabilities as may be prescribed by the Minister" (N.A.A. 1948, s.29(1)). The guiding principle is to ensure that all handicapped persons should have the maximum opportunity of sharing in, and contributing to, the life of the community, so that their capacities are realised to the full, their self-confidence developed, and their social contacts strengthened (*Ministry of Health Circular No. 87* (1948, para. 60). The 1948 Act (s.64(1)) defines "blind person" as "a person so blind as to be unable to perform any work for which eyesight is essential." It does not expand upon the meaning of the other disabilities listed in section 29(1).

In addition to the power in section 29(1), there is a duty (under s.29(2)) to exercise the powers in relation to persons ordinarily resident in the area of the local authority "to such extent as the Minister may direct." The welfare arrangements are to be carried into effect in accordance with a scheme (s.29(3)). The scheme is to be made by the local authority and submitted to the Minister. It comes into force when approved by him (N.A.A. 1948, s.34(2)). Not later than the date on which the scheme is submitted to the Minister the local authority must send a copy to the council of each county district in the county. Before approving the scheme the Minister must take into consideration any representations made by any of the councils within one month of the date of submission to the Minister (s.34(3)). The Minister may approve the scheme in its original form, or with modifications (s.34(4)). A scheme may be varied or revoked by a subsequent scheme (s.34(5)). Where it appears to the Minister that by reason of a change of circumstances it is expedient that a scheme should be varied, he may require the local authority to submit within a specified time a varying scheme for his approval. If the local authority fails to comply, the Minister may himself make the varying scheme (s.34(7)). Where no scheme is in force for the exercise of powers under section 29 which the local authority is under a duty to exercise, the Minister may require the authority to submit a scheme within a specified time, and if it fails to do so, or submits a scheme unsuitable for approval either with or without modification, the Minister may make the scheme himself. The particulars required by the Minister in a scheme are set out in Ministry of Health Circular No. 87 (1948).

The arrangements that a local authority may make under section 29 of the 1948 Act include the provision of workshops and hostels, so that disabled persons may be engaged in suitable work and may have somewhere to live whilst so engaged (s.29(4)(c)).

In addition to this provision, there is provision also in the Disabled Persons (Employment) Act 1958. Section 3 of this gives local authorities the power to provide sheltered employment for registered persons who are seriously disabled. It provides (s.3(2)) that this power is "in lieu of any power or duty" of the authority to make arrangements for the same purposes under section 29 of the 1948 Act. For the relationships between the two provisions, the Schedule to the 1958 Act (para. 3) may be consulted.

The Health and Social Services and Social Security Adjudications Act 1983 enables a local authority which provides services under section 29 of the 1948 Act to recover such charge, if any, as it considers reasonable (s.17(1), (2)). However, if a person avails himself of a service under section 29 and satisfies the authority that his means are insufficient for it to be "reasonably practicable" for him to pay for the service the amount which he would otherwise be obliged to pay, "the authority shall not require him to pay more . . . than it appears to them that it is reasonably practicable for him to pay" (s.17(3)). It should be noted that the onus of proof is upon the disabled person, a position which it is somewhat hard to justify. It is further provided that charges may be recovered summarily as a civil debt (s.17(4)).

Despite the existence of these welfare services, a major criticism of the provisions of the 1948 Act is its failure to provide sufficient by way of supportive services to enable care to be provided for the elderly or handicapped at home. Later legislative provisions have made some attempt to plug this gap.

The Health Services and Public Health Act 1968 contains some provisions of this nature. Section 12 empowers a local health authority to make arrangements for the purpose of the prevention of illness, for the care of persons suffering from illness and for the aftercare of persons who have been so suffering. Included is the provision of "centres or other facilities for training" such persons or "keeping them suitably occupied" (s.12(1)(b)). In pursuing the development of community-based services for elderly and physically handicapped people, the 1968 Act also imposes a duty on local health authorities "to provide on such a scale as is adequate for the needs of their area, or to arrange for the provision on such a scale as is so adequate of, home help for households where such help is required owing to the presence of a person who is suffering from illness, lying-in, an expectant mother, aged, handicapped as a result of having suffered from illness or by congenital deformity or a child" under school-leaving age (s.13). It should be noted that the authorities are under a duty: in earlier legislation (National Health Service Act 1946, s.29) there was merely a power to provide domestic help. There are default powers in the Minister in cases where the local health authority fails in its duty. He may order the authority to "discharge such of their functions, in such manner and within such time or times, as may be specified in the order." If the authority still fails to comply, the Minister may, in addition to invoking remedies of administrative law, transfer to himself such of the functions of the authority as he thinks fit (s.57(3) of the National Health Service Act 1946, applicable to the 1968 Act by virtue of s.43(4) and Sched. 2).

Local health authorities are also given the power under the 1968 Act (s.13) to provide or arrange for the provision of laundry facilities for households for which home help is, or can be, provided. It is not accordingly a pre-condition of laundry facilities being provided that home help is also given. A local health authority may, with the Minister's approval, recover such charges, if any, as it thinks reasonable from the persons using a home help or laundry facilities (H.S. & P.H.A. 1968, s.13(2)).

There is also in section 45 of the 1968 Act, a general power vested in local authorities to promote the welfare of old people. The authority may use as its agent any voluntary organisation "having for its sole or principal objects, or among its principal objects, the promotion of the welfare of old people" (s.45(3)). The authority may charge the old person for its services whatever is considered reasonable (H. & S.S. & S.S.A.A. 1983, s.17(1) and (2)(*b*) replacing H.S. & P.H.A. 1968, s.45(2)).

VII. *The Chronically Sick and Disabled Persons Act 1970*

A landmark in the law relating to the physically handicapped is the Chronically Sick and Disabled Persons Act 1970. It was the patchy provision of services for physically handicapped people prior to 1970 which prompted Alf Morris to introduce the private members' bill which became the 1970 Act. Section 29 of the National Assistance Act 1948 had given local authorities the power to promote the welfare of the disabled. Many local authorities took a rather limited view of their responsibilities under this section. The resulting concern facilitated the passage of the 1970 Act. The Act was hailed as "a charter for the disabled." The Act has been a profound disappointment. It has created expectations which have not, and perhaps cannot in the current economic climate, be fulfilled. Much of the Act is anyway only likely to benefit the disabled in indirect ways: eight of the 28 provisions are designed to ensure the representation of the interests of the disabled on governmental or advisory committees; a further six require housing authorities and those concerned with public buildings, universities and schools "to have regard to" the special needs of the chronically sick and disabled, or to make provision as to access, parking or sanitary conveniences "so far as it is in the circumstances both practicable and reasonable" for the disabled. The end results of such legislation are not necessarily productive.

At the time the Act was passed, there was concern that many of the disabled were slipping through the net. Accordingly, section 1 of the Act imposes a duty on all local authorities with responsibilities (the Act says "functions") under section 29 of the 1948 Act to inform themselves of the number of persons to whom that section applies. It does not provide for compulsory registration of disabled persons. Some advocated this. Many, however, including many disabled persons, would regard that as a retrograde and unnecessary step. Section 1 also imposes a duty on authorities to publish information of the services provided and to ensure that a disabled person is informed of any of those services which "in the opinion of the authority is relevant to his needs" (s.1(2)(*b*)).

The main provisions of the Act of direct assistance to those in need are those dealing with vehicles (ss.20 and 21) and with welfare services generally. The Act enabled regulations governing road traffic to be relaxed to meet special needs (for example it enabled small electrically-driven cars provided for some child victims of the thalidomide disaster to be used legally on the pavement (s.20(1)(*a*)). It also provided for special badges for display on cars used by disabled drivers and passengers. Cars with badges are exempt from some parking regulations (C.S. & D.P.A. 1970, s.21: see also the Disabled Persons (Badges for Motor Vehicles) Regulations 1982 (S.I. 1982 No. 1740).

The central provision in the Act is in section 2. This provides that where a local authority is satisfied that it is necessary in order to meet the needs of a relevant person to make arrangements for all or any of the following matters, it must do so. These matters are:

(a) the provision of practical assistance for that person in the home;

(b) the provision for that person of, or assistance to that person in obtaining, wireless, television, library or similar recreational facilities;

(c) the provision for that person of lectures, games, outings or other recreational facilities outside his home or assistance to that person in taking educational facilities available to him;

(d) the provision for that person of facilities for, or assistance in, travelling to and from his home for the purpose of participating in any services provided under arrangements made by the authority;

(e) the provision of assistance for that person in arranging for the carrying out of any works of adaptation in his home or the provision of any additional facilities designed to secure his greater safety, comfort or convenience;

(f) facilitating the taking of holidays by that person;

(g) the provision of meals for that person whether in his home or elsewhere;

(h) the provision for that person of, or assistance to that person in obtaining, a telephone and any special equipment necessary to enable him to use a telephone.

The Act also provides (in s.4) that buildings to which the public are admitted shall "in so far as it is in the circumstances both practicable and reasonable" make provision for the needs of members of the public who are disabled visiting the building. There is a specific and separate provision (in s.8) applying to universities, schools, colleges and other educational establishments.

The Chronically Sick and Disabled Persons Act applies to the sick and disabled of all ages. It applies to those whose handicaps are the result of some mental disorder as well as to those whose disability is of a physical nature.

It is clear that it can only be enforced in one way, namely by the default procedure set out in section 36 of the National Assistance Act 1948. The aggrieved person must accordingly make representations to the Minister who may declare the authority to be in default. He is then to direct the authority to discharge its functions. If it fails to do so, he may make an order transferring to himself such of the authority's functions as he thinks fit. As Wade (1982) observes this "is suitable for dealing with a general breakdown of some public service caused by a local authority's default, but it is quite unsuitable as a remedy for defaults in individual cases." But the courts have held the default procedure to be exhaustive (*Wyatt* v. *Hillingdon L.B.C.*, 1978). Geoffrey Lane L.J. in the Court of Appeal said of the 1970 Act:

> "A statute such as this which is dealing with the distribution of benefits—or, to put it perhaps more accurately, comforts to the sick and disabled—does not in its very nature give rise to an action by the disappointed sick person. It seems to me quite extraordinary that if the local authority, as is alleged here, provided, for example, two hours less home help than the sick person considered herself entitled to that that can amount to a breach of statutory duty which will permit the sick person to claim a sum of monetary damages by way of breach of statutory duty. It seems to me that eminently that is the sort of situation where precisely the remedy provided by section 36 of the Act of 1948 is appropriate and an action in damages is not appropriate."

These sentiments, harsh though they are, are consistent with orthodox legal thinking. They mean that the courts are barred to aggrieved persons, where a default procedure exists. It should, however, be noted that legal remedies are available where the local authority acts outside the scope of its powers (*ultra vires*), in which case a declaration or injunction might be sought or where the local authority fetters its own discretion by invoking over-rigid policies which do not enable it to consider cases on their merits (see *Att.-Gen. ex rel. Tilley* v. *Wandsworth L.B.C.*, 1981). Furthermore, where representations are made to the Minister, it is clear that he has a duty as well as a power: he cannot use his discretion to frustrate the policy of the Act. Were he to be allowed to do so he would be rendering nugatory a safeguard provided by the Act (*Padfield* v. *Minister of Agriculture, Fisheries and Food*, 1968).

The 1970 Act has not worked (*Morris*, 1982) and further reforms may be expected in the near future. In particular it is anticipated that legislation may be proposed to outlaw discrimination against the disabled.

Welfare services are also provided for in two other Acts.

VIII. *The National Health Service Act 1977*

A small part of this Act is concerned with prevention, care and aftercare services of local social services authorities. Provision is made for local authorities to make arrangements for the purpose of the prevention of illness, for the care of people suffering from illness and for the aftercare of people who have been suffering from illness. These arrangements are subject to the Secretary of State's approval and to the extent that he may direct shall include:

(a) the provision, equipment and maintenance of residential accommodation for the care of people with a view to the prevention of illness, the care of people who are ill, and their aftercare;

(b) the provision, equipment and maintenance of centres and other facilities for the training or occupation of people within the above categories;

(c) the provision of ancillary or supplemental services (Sched. 8, para. 2(1)).

The local authority may recover such charge, if any, as it considers reasonable for any of these services (the H. & S.S. & S.S.A. 1983, s.17(2)(c)).

IX. *The Health and Social Services and Social Security Adjudications Act 1983*

The Residential Homes Act of 1980 provided (s.8) for district councils (*i.e.* councils of county districts) to have the power to make arrangements to provide meals and recreation (not further defined) for old people in their homes or elsewhere. This provision is repealed by Schedule 10 of the 1983 Act, although section 17 of that Act enables authorities to charge for services under section 8 of the 1980 Act! However, Schedule 9, Part II of th 1983 Act, re-enacts substantially the same provisions as the repealed 1980 section 8, and section 17 of the 1983 enables authorities to charge for services provided under Schedule 9, Pt. II, para. 1.

The upshot of this charade, a piece of lunacy dating from the last week of the first Thatcher administration, is that district councils may make arrangements for the provision of meals and recreation for old people in their homes or elsewhere and may employ as their agent any voluntary organisation whose activities consist in or include the provision of such services. District councils may assist a voluntary organisation by contributing to its funds, by permitting it to use premises belonging to the council on such terms as may be agreed and by making available furniture, vehicles or equipment (by way of gift, loan or otherwise) and the services of any staff who are employed by the council in connection with the premises or other things which the voluntary organisation is permitted to use. A voluntary organisation is defined to exclude a public or local authority and must not operate for profit.

12. Nursing Homes and other Residential Homes

I. *Nursing Homes*

The law governing nursing homes is found in the Registered Homes Act 1984 which replaces the Nursing Homes Act 1975, as amended by the Health Services Act 1980 and the H. & S.S. & S.S.A. 1983.

A nursing home is defined (Registered Homes Act 1984, s.21) as any premises used, or intended to be used,

   (a) for the reception of, and provision of nursing for, persons suffering from any sickness, injury or infirmity;

   (b) for the reception of pregnant women, or of women immediately after childbirth (maternity homes); and

   (c) for the provision of all or any of the following services:

      (i) the carrying out of surgical procedures under anaesthesia;

     (ii) the termination of pregnancies;

    (iii) endoscopy;

    (iv) haemodialysis or peritoneal dialysis;

     (v) treatment (including diagnosis) by specially controlled techniques. (See s.21(6)).

A specially controlled technique is "any technique of medicine or surgery (including cosmetic surgery)" specified in regulations to be made by the Secretary of State. He is to specify any technique which he is satisfied may "create a hazard for persons treated by means of it or for the staff of any premises where the technique is used" (R.H.A. 1984, s.21(4)).

The following are defined so as not to be nursing homes:

(a) hospitals maintained or controlled by a Government department, a local authority or body constituted by special Act of Parliament or incorporated by Royal Charter;

(b) mental nursing homes;

(c) sanatoria provided at schools and other educational establishments and used solely by persons in attendance or by staff or their families (in a wide, popular rather than technical sense);

(d) First Aid or treatment rooms at factory premises, sports and show grounds and places of public entertainment;

(e) doctors', dentists' and chiropodists' surgeries and premises used for occupational health facilities;

(f) any premises used wholly or mainly (that is, more than half the time: *Fawcett Properties* v. *Bucks C.C.*, 1961) as a private dwelling.

(g) any other premises excepted from the definition of nursing homes by regulations, as yet unmade, issued by the Secretary of State.

Registration

Nursing homes must be registered with the Secretary of State (s.23(3)). Any person who carries on a nursing home without being registered commits an offence (s.23(11)). The certificate of registration must be "kept affixed in a conspicuous place in the home"; failure to do so is also an offence (s.23(6)). It is also an offence to hold out premises as a nursing home or maternity home with intent to deceive unless registration has been effected under the Act in respect of the premises as such a home (R.H.A. 1984, s.24).

To obtain a certificate of registration the health authority, to which the Secretary of State has delegated the office, may require information to be furnished as to the following matters (see S.I. 1981 No. 932, reg.3(2) and Sched. 2).

(1) The full name and address, and professional or technical qualifications (if any) of the applicant.

(2) Where the application is made by a company, society, association or body, the address of its registered office or principal place of business and the full names and address and technical qualifications (if any) of the directors or partners.

(3) The address of any other home or of any residential home for mentally disordered persons or of any disabled persons' or old persons' home within the meaning of the 1983 Act in which the applicant has or had a business interest and the nature and extent of his interest.

(4) The situation of the home and its form of construction.

(5) The accommodation available, and the equipment and facilities provided or to be provided in the home.

(6) The date on which the home was established or is to be established.

(7) Whether any other business is or will be carried on in the same premises as the home.

(8) The type of nursing home (*e.g.* mental, maternity, clinic catering for day-patients only).

(9) The number of patients (excluding staff) for whom it is proposed to be used, distinguishing between different categories of patients and indicating the age-range of patients in each category.

(10) The full names, ages, qualifications and experience of persons employed or proposed to be employed in the management of the home and whether they are or will be resident in the home.

(11) The arrangements for the management and control of the home.

(12) The full names and qualifications of any resident or non-resident employed medical practitioners.

(13) The full names and (where appropriate) qualifications and grades of the nursing and other professional, technical, administrative and ancillary staff (other than staff included in (12)) employed or proposed to be employed in the home, distinguishing between resident and non-resident staff.

(14) The details of arrangements made or proposed to be made in pursuance of any matter relating to the provision of facilities and services (see r.10 below).

(15) The arrangements made for the supply of blood and blood products.

(16) The arrangements made for the provision of pathology and radiology services.

It should be noted that the provisions of the Rehabilitation of Offenders Act 1974 relating to spent convictions (s.4(1)), questions about previous convictions (s.4(2)) and convictions as a ground for dismissing or excluding a person from an office (s.4(3)(*b*)) do not apply in this context (see Rehabilitation of Offenders Act 1974 (Exemptions) Order (S.I. 1975 No. 1023)).

An application for registration must be in writing, sent or delivered to the health authority and accompanied by the requisite fee (S.I. 1981 No. 932, reg.3).

Registration may be refused. Section 25 of the 1984 Act provides that the Secretary of State may refuse to register an applicant if satisfied that

    (a) the applicant, an employee or proposed employee is not a fit person, whether by reason of age or otherwise to carry on or be employed;

    (b) the home is not fit to be used owing to its situation, construction, state of repair, accommodation, staffing or equipment;

    (c) the home is, or premises used in connection therewith are, used or proposed to be used, for purposes which are improper or undesirable;

    (d) the home is, or premises used in connection therewith consist of, or include works executed in contravention of section 12(1) of the Health Services Act 1976 (which controls the construction of hospital building) or of any term contained in an authorisation under section 13 of that Act.

    (e) the home is not, or will not be, in the charge of a person who is either a registered medical practitioner or qualified nurse or, in the case of a maternity home, a certified midwife.

A home may also be registered subject to conditions and these may be varied.

The registration of a nursing home may be cancelled by the Secretary of State on any of the grounds which would have entitled him to refuse an application for registration (in the case of (e) above the registration is not to be cancelled before the expiration of three months beginning with the service of notice on the person concerned), or where the person concerned has been convicted of an offence against the provisions of the Acts or any other person has been convicted of such an offence in respect of the home, or on the ground that the annual fee in respect of the home has not been paid. Registration may also be cancelled for offences against regulations made under the Acts (R.H.A. 1984, s.28).

The 1983 Act (Sched. 4, Pt. II, para. 32) now provides detailed procedures for cancellation of registration. There is an urgent procedure and an ordinary procedure.

The *urgent procedure* requires an application by the Secretary of State to a Justice of the Peace. If it appears to the J.P. that "there will be a serious risk to the life, health or well-being of the patients in the home" unless an order is made, he may make the order. This will have the effect of cancelling the registration, varying a condition or imposing an additional condition on the person concerned (the Secretary of State will have asked for one of these three orders). The application is *ex parte* and must be supported by a written statement of the Secretary of State's reasons for making the application. The order and a statement of the Secretary of State's reasons must be served on the person registered in respect of the home as soon as practicable after the making of the order.

The *ordinary procedure* requires the Secretary of State to give an applicant notice including reasons of a proposal to refuse his application, to cancel the registration, to vary any condition or impose any new one. A notice must state that within 14 days of service of the notice any person on whom it is served may in writing require the Secretary of State to give him an opportunity to make representations to him concerning any matter which that person wishes to dispute. The matter in dispute cannot then be determined until representations have been made, the period for making representations has elapsed, or the person concerned has failed to make representations within the reasonable period allowed him by the Secretary of State. Representations may be made either orally or in writing. If oral representations are requested, the Secretary of State has to give the person concerned an opportunity of appearing before and being heard by a person appointed by the Secretary of State.

If after this procedure the Secretary of State decides to adopt the proposal, he must serve notice in writing of his decision on any person on whom he was required to serve notice of the proposal. This must include a note explaining the right of appeal. If an appeal is brought, the decision cannot take effect until it is determined or abandoned, otherwise, the decision cannot effect until a period of 28 days has elapsed after service of notice of the decision.

Appeals lie to a Registered Homes Tribunal against decisions of the Secretary of State and orders made under the urgent procedure by a J.P. Notice in writing must be given to the Secretary of State within 28 days of service of notice of the decision or order. The tribunal's powers are to confirm the decision or order or direct that it shall cease to have effect, to vary conditions, direct that they shall cease to have effect or impose conditions in respect of the home. The Secretary of State must comply with any directions of a tribunal. (See s.34 of the 1984 Act).

Records

The 1981 Regulations require the person registered to maintain a record "in the form of a register" of all patients in the home. This is to include:

  (a) the name, address and date of birth of the patient;
  (b) the name and address of next of kin or person authorised to act on the patient's behalf;
  (c) the name and address of the patient's medical practitioner;
  (d) the date on which the patient entered and left the home;
  (e) if the patient is transferred to hospital, the date and reasons for the transfer and the name of the hospital concerned;
  (f) if the patient dies in the home, the date, time and cause of death (reg.6(1)); (The health authority must be notified of any death within 24 hours, extended in the case of weekends, public holidays and bank holidays (reg.7).)
  (g) a record of nursing staff employed at the home (reg.6(8)).

In the case of maternity homes, additional particulars are required (date and time of delivery, sex of child, name and qualifications of person who delivered patient, date and time of any miscarriages, date when child born in home left it, date and time of any death of a child born to a patient). A separate record of surgical operations must be kept. All these records must be retained for a minimum of one year from the date of the last entry in the register.

The person registered is also required to maintain a "case record" in respect of each patient to include the following particulars:

  (a) an adequate daily statement of the patient's health and condition; and
  (b) a note of any investigations and details of surgical operations carried out and any treatment given.

In the case of a maternity home, a case record in respect of each child born must be kept, to include the child's weight and condition, a daily statement of the child's health and details of certain paediatric examinations.

Facilities and services

The 1981 Regulations lay down the facilities and services that "having regard to the size of the home and the number, age, sex and condition of the patients" the person registered must provide (r.10). These are:

(a) adequate (meaning sufficient and suitable) professional, technical, ancillary and other staff;

(b) adequate accommodation and space including, where appropriate, day-room facilities;

(c) adequate furniture, bedding, curtains and, where necessary, suitable screens and floor covering;

(d) adequate medical, surgical and nursing equipment and treatment facilities;

(e) adequate sanitary facilities;

(f) adequate light, heating and ventilation;

(g) all parts of the home must be kept in good structural repair, clean and reasonably decorated;

(h) there must be adequate fire precautions;

(i) adequate kitchen equipment;

(j) adequate food;

(k) appropriate laundering facilities;

(l) adequate arrangements for the disposal of swabs, soiled dressings, etc.;

(m) adequate arrangements for patients to receive medical and dental services;

(n) adequate arrangements for recording, safe keeping, handling and disposal of drugs;

(o) adequate arrangements for the prevention of infection, toxic conditions and the spread of infection in the home;

(p) adequate arrangements where appropriate for the training or occupation and recreation of patients and play and education facilities for children;

(q) adequate precautions against the risk of accident;

(r) adequate facilities for any person authorised to interview any patient in the home;

(s) a telephone service.

It is an offence to fail to comply with the regulation requiring these facilities and services (reg. 11(3), (4)). The offence is punishable by fine but more significantly may lead to the cancellation of registration. Where the Secretary of State considers that the person registered has failed or is failing to conduct the home in accordance with the regulations, he may serve a notice specifying in what respect there is failure and what action should be taken so as to comply with the regulation and within what period action should be taken.

Inspection

The 1981 Regulations (reg. 9) provide for inspections of nursing homes on such occasions and at such intervals as he may decide but in any case not less than twice in every period of 12 months. To this end, authorised persons may enter and inspect any premises which are used, or which he reasonably believes to be used, as a nursing home and in the course of such inspection may require the production of records. He may require the person registered to furnish such information in relation to the nursing home as may reasonably be required for the purposes of inspection. However, a person who is not a medical officer may not inspect any clinical record relating to a patient in a home. (See reg. 8).

II. *Mental Nursing Homes*

A mental nursing home is defined by section 22 of the Registered Homes Act 1984. "Mental nursing home" means any premises used, or intended to be used, for the reception of, and the provision of nursing or other medical treatment (including care, habilitation and rehabilitation under medical supervision) for one or more mentally disordered patients (*i.e.* persons suffering, or appearing to be suffering from mental disorder), whether exclusively or in common with other persons. Mental nursing homes must be distinguised from N.H.S. hospitals, accommodation provided by a local authority and used as a hospital and special hospitals, as well as from disabled and old persons' homes. The few remaining voluntary hospitals for the mentally disordered do, however, come within the ambit of "mental nursing home."

As with nursing homes, mental nursing homes must be registered (R.H.A. 1984, s.23). The registration provisions are as for nursing homes (*q.v.*) with one addition. If a home is to take patients who are subject to compulsory detention (see p.130), it must be registered in a separate part of the register (s.23(5)(*b*)). The 1983 Act (Sched. 4, Pt. II, para. 26) created a new offence of holding out premises as a mental nursing home when registration has not been effected. (See now 1984 Act, s.24).

Registration may be refused if the applicants or premises are unfit (R.H.A. 1984, s.25). (The details are broadly as for nursing homes, *q.v.*) Registration can also be cancelled in certain circumstances (s.28) (again the details are similar to those for nursing homes, *q.v.*). If a home has compulsory patients in it when registration is cancelled or the registered person dies, the registration continues in force for two months to enable alternative arrangements for them to be made (N.H.A. 1975, s.36). The procedures (urgent and ordinary) for cancellation of registration are as for nursing homes (*q.v.*).

Mental nursing homes, as well as places suspected to be operating as such, are subject to inspection on behalf of the Secretary of State (R.H.A. 1984, s.35). Inspectors may visit and interview in private any patient residing in the home for the purpose of investigating any complaint as to his treatment made by, or on behalf of, the patient or in any case where the inspector has reasonable cause to believe that the patient is not receiving proper care. If the inspector is a doctor, he may also examine the patient in private and may require the production of, and inspect, any medical records relating to the patient's treatment in home (R.H.A. 1984, s.35(2)). It is an offence to refuse to allow premises to be inspected or otherwise to infere with or obstruct an inspection, interview or examination (s.35(5), (6)). Inspection must take place at least twice in every period of 12 months (S.I. 1981 No. 932, reg.9).

III. *Residential Care Homes*

The law governing residential care homes is now found in the Registered Homes Act 1984.

A "residential care home" is an establishment which provides or intended to provide, whether for reward or not, residential accommodation with both board and personal care for persons in need of this by reason of old age, disablement, past or present dependence on alcohol or drugs or past or present mental disorder (s.1(1)).

There is a requirement for registration and it is an offence not to register, punishable by a small fine. (See s.2). Establishments with less than four residents are exempt from this requirement. (s.1(4)). So are nursing homes and mental nursing homes (they may register if they wish), hospitals, mental hospitals, community homes and voluntary homes for children, other children's homes (within the meaning of the Children's Homes Act 1982), schools other than independent schools for less than 50 children which are also not approved under the Education Act 1981, s.11(3)(*a*), universities and their halls, and "any establishment managed or provided by a government department or local authority or by any authority or body constituted by an Act of Parliament or incorporated by Royal Charter." (s.1(5)).

The requirement to register extends beyond managers where they are not in control of the home to the person who is in control. (s.3). The certificate of registration will state the maximum number of persons who may be resident. This condition, and any others, must be complied with. The certificate of registration must be affixed in a conspicuous place in the home.

In one circumstance, a home may be carried on by a person who is not registered. Where the only person registered dies his personal representatives, his widow (including someone who has lived with the deceased as his wife for not less than six months) or any other relative (very broadly defined to include relationships by affinity, illegitimate relationships and persons with whom the registered person has been ordinarily residing for a period of at least five years) may carry on the home for four weeks or such longer period as the registration authority may sanction. (s.6).

Registration may be refused by the registration authority if satisfied that the personnel involved or the home is not fit or "the way in which it is intended to carry on or the home is such as not to provide services or facilities reasonably required." (s.9). Registration may be cancelled on the same grounds as well as upon conviction of various offences and failure to pay the registration fee. Both urgent and ordinary procedures for cancellation of registration are provided for. These are as for nursing homes and were discussed in detail earlier in this chapter (*q.v.*).

Residential care homes are to be subject to regular inspection.

Regulations as yet unissued will provide how often such inspections are to take place. Both the Secretary of State and the registration authority may appoint inspectors.

The 1984 Act also gives the Secretary of State power to make regulations as to the conduct of residential care homes on such matters as (a) facilities and services; (b) numbers and qualifications of staff; (c) records; (d) making provision for children to receive a religious upbringing. (See s.16).

IV. *Registered Homes Tribunals*

The tribunal is to consist of a legal chairman and two experts with experience in social work, medicine, nursing or midwifery or "such other experience as the Lord President of the Council considers suitable" (R.H.A. 1984, s.40.) If the appeal relates solely to registration under the Registered Homes Act 1984, it is to include a registered medical practitioner and a qualified nurse (where the appeal relates to registration of a maternity home, a qualified midwife).

The Secretary of State may by statutory instrument, make rules as to the practice and procedure to be followed in Registered Homes Tribunals. (See s.43 of the 1984 Act).

Bibliography of References and Further Reading

Chapter 1

Cawson, P., *Community Homes—A Study of Residential Staff* (H.M.S.O., 1978).

Children's Legal Centre, *Locked-up in Care* (C.L.C., 1982).

Crowther, M.A., *The Workhouse System 1834–1929* (Batsford, 1981).

Curtis Report, The. *The Report of the Care of Children Committee* Cmd. 6922 (H.M.S.O., 1946).

Davis, A., *The Residential Solution* (Tavistock, 1981).

DHSS, *Intermediate Treatment—A Guide for the Regional Planning of New Forms of Treatment for Children in Trouble* (H.M.S.O., 1972).

DHSS, *Youth Treatment Centres* (H.M.S.O., 1971).

DHSS, Local Authority Circular 1/75, *Secure Accommodation in Community Homes* (DHSS, 1975).

DHSS, Local Authority Circular 77/1, *Children and Young Persons Act 1969* (DHSS, 1977).

DHSS, Local Authority Circular 83/8, *Criminal Justice Act 1982, s. 25—Restriction of Liberty—The Secure Accommodation Regulations 1983*.

Hoggett, B., *Parents and Children* (Sweet & Maxwell, 1981).

Home Office, *Press Release, The Times*, May 24, 1983.

Home Office, Welsh Office, DHSS, *Young Offenders* Cmnd. 8045 (H.M.S.O., 1980).

Home Office Circular 9/1480, *Detention Centres—General Revision of Committal Areas; Introduction of More Rigorous Regimes at Two Centres* (H.O.C., 1980).

House of Commons Debates, Vol. 22, ser. 102, cols. 524 *et seq.* (1982).

House of Lords Debates, Vol. 431, col. 971, Lord Elton.

Ingleby Report, The. *Report of the Committee on Children and Young Persons* Cmnd. 1141 (H.M.S.O., 1960).

Leeding, A., *Leeding's Child Care Manual for Social Workers* (Butterworths, 1980).

McEwan, J. A., "In Search of Juvenile Justice—The Criminal Justice Act 1982" [1983] J.S.W.L. 112–117.

McEwan, J. A., "The Criminal Justice Act—Justice Welfare or Confusion?" (1983) M.L.R. 25–30.

Report of the Departmental Committee on Young Offenders Cmd. 2831 (H.M.S.O., 1927).

Shearer, A., *Handicapped Children in Residential Care* (Bedford Square Press, 1980).

Statistics of Education, Vol. 1 (H.M.S.O.), 1961 Table 17; 1966 Table 35; 1971 Table 28; 1976 Table 23; 1977 Table 26; 1979 Table 25.

The Williams Report, Caring for People; Staffing Residential Homes (Allen & Unwin, 1967).

Warnock, M., *Report of the Committee of Enquiry into the Education of Handicapped Children and Young People* Cmnd. 7212 (H.M.S.O., 1978).

Chapter 2

Adcock, M., and White, R., "Care Orders or the Assumption of Parental Rights—the Long-Term Effects" [1980] J.S.W.L. 257.

Aldgate, J., "Advantages of Residential Care" [1978] *Adoption & Fostering*, 29–33.

Bevan, H. K., and Parry, M., *The Children Act 1975* (Butterworths, 1979).

Bottoms, A., "The Suspended Sentence in England and Wales 1967–1978" (1981) 21 B.J.Crim. 1.

British Agencies for Adoption and Fostering (formerly A.B.A.F.A.), *The Rights of Children* (1980).

DHSS, *Children in Care in England and Wales* (Information Unit, 1982).

DHSS, Leaflet Nos. 1 and 2. *For Parents and Guardians whose Children are received into Care* (1977).

DHSS, Scottish Education Department and Welsh Office, *Guide to Fostering Practice* (H.M.S.O., 1976).

Eekelaar, J., "What are Parental Rights?" (1973) 89 L.Q.R. 210.

Family Rights Group, *Problems over Access* (London, 1983).

Feldman, L., *Care Proceedings* (Oyez, 1978).

Freeman, M. D. A., Controlling Local Authorities in Child Care Cases—A. *v.* Liverpool City Council Revisited (1982) J.P. Vol. 146, pp. 188, 202.

Freeman, M. D. A., *The Child Care and Foster Children Act 1980* (Sweet & Maxwell, 1980).

Freeman, M. D. A., "The Legal Battlefield of Care" [1982] C.L.P. 117.

Hall, J., "The Waning of Parental Rights" (1972) 31 C.L.J. 248.

Hoggett, B., *Parents and Children* (Sweet & Maxwell, 1981).

Home Office Circular 91/1977, *The Certificates of Unruly Character Conditions Order* (1977).

Home Office, Circular 20/1971 *Children and Young Persons Act 1969: Section 24(5), The Children and Young Persons* (Definition of Independent Persons) Regulations 1971.

Lowe, N. V., and White, R., *Wards of Court* (Butterworths, 1979).

Lyon, C. M., "A Voluntary Trap—Children in Care under s.1 Children Act 1948" [1979] *Liverpool Law Rev.* 97–113.

McEwan, J. A., "Commentary on Vicar of Writtle v. Essex County Council" [1980] J.S.W.L. 48–52.

McEwan, J. A., "In Search of Juvenile Justice—The Criminal Justice Act 1982" [1983] J.S.W.L. 112–117.

McEwan, J. A., "The Criminal Justice—Justice Welfare or Confusion" (1983) M.L.R. 25–30.

Maidment, S., "Assumption of Parental Rights" in H. Geach and E. Szwed (eds.) *Providing Civil Justice for the Child* (Arnold, 1983).

Maidment, S., "The Fragmentation of Parental Rights and Children in Care" [1981] J.S.W.L. 21–35.

Page, R., and Clark, G. *Who Cares?* (N.C.B., 1979).

Rowe, J., and Lambert, L., *Children Who Wait* (A.B.A.F.A., 1973).

Sinclair, R., "The Functions of Reviews On Children in Care" (1983) 7 *Social Work, Medicine, The Law No. 2,* 43.

Smith, R., *Children and the Courts* (Sweet & Maxwell, 1979).

Thomson, J. M., "Local Authorities and Parental Rights" (1974) 90 L.Q.R. 310, (1975) 91 L.Q.R. 14.

Chapter 3

Cawson, P., *Community Homes: A Study of Residential Staff* (H.M.S.O., 1978).

Crossman, R., *The Diaries of a Cabinet Minister* (Hamish Hamilton & Jonathan Cape, 1977) Vol. 3, pp. 409, 418.

Curtis Report, The. *The Report of the Care and Children Committee* Cmd. 6922 (H.M.S.O., 1946).

DHSS, Advisory Council on Child Care, *Care and treatment in a planned environment* (H.M.S.O., 1970).

DHSS, *Children Referred to Closed Units* (H.M.S.O., 1979).

DHSS Circular No. 78/1972, *Children and Young Persons Act 1969; The Community Homes Regulations* (1972).

DHSS, *Legal and Professional Aspects of the Use of Secure Accommodation for Children in Care* (DHSS, 1981).

DHSS, Letter to Directors of Social Services, *Secure Accommodation Regulations—Commencement Arrangements*, April 5, 1983.

DHSS, Local Authority Circular 1/1975, *Secure Accommodation in Community Homes* (DHSS, 1975).

DHSS Local Authority Circular 77/1, *Children and Young Persons Act 1969—Intermediate Treatment* (1977).

DHSS Local Authority Circular 83/8, *Criminal Justice Act 1982, s. 25—Restriction of Liberty—The Secure Accommodation Regulations 1983* (1983).

DHSS, *Report of a Survey of long-stay hospital accommodation for Children* (H.M.S.O., 1970).

Home Office Circular No. 159/1971, *Detention Centres*—The report of the Advisory Council on the Penal System (Home Office, 1971).

Home Office, Welsh Office, DHSS, *Young Offenders* Cmnd. 8045 (H.M.S.O., 1980).

King, R., Raynes, N., and Tizard, J., *Patterns of Residential Care* (Routledge and Kegal Paul, 1971).

Millham, S., Bullock, R., and Hosie, K., *Locking up Children— Secure Provision within the Child Care System* (Saxon House, Farnborough, 1978).

National Health Service, *Annual Report of the Hospital Advisory Service*, to the Secretary of State for Social Services and the Secretary of State for Wales for the year 1972 (H.M.S.O., 1973), para. 159.

Oswin, M., *Children Living in Long-Stay Hospitals* (Spastics International Medical Publications, Heinemann, 1978).

P.S.S.C., *Residential Care Reviewed*, the report of the Residential Care Working Group, incorporating "Daily Living—Questions for Staff" (1977).

Parliamentary All Party Penal Affairs Group, *Young Offenders—A Strategy for the Future* (H.M.S.O., 1982).

Report of the Committee of Enquiry into Allegations of Ill-treatment of Patients and Other Irregularities at the Ely Hospital, Cardiff Cmnd. 3875 (H.M.S.O., 1969).

Shearer, A., *Handicapped Children in Residential Care—A Study of Policy Failure* (Bedford Square Press, 1980).

Smith, R., *Children and the Courts* (Sweet & Maxwell, 1979).

Warnock, M., *Report of the Committee of Enquiry into the Education of Handicapped Children and Young People* Cmnd. 7212 (H.M.S.O., 1978).

Wills, D., *Spare the Child* (Penguin, 1971).

Chapter 4

DHSS, *Community Care* (1980).

Green Paper, *Recommendations on Local Government Finance* Cmnd. 6813 (H.M.S.O., 1977).

Hoggett, B., *Parents and Children* (Sweet & Maxwell, 1981).

Holman, R., *Inequality in Child Care* (C.P.A.G., 1980).

Home Office Circular No. 285/1970, *Children and Young Persons Act 1969—Parental Contributions* (Home Office, 1970).

Layfield Committee, *The Committee of Inquiry into Local Government Finance* Cmnd. 6453 (H.M.S.O., 1974).

Lister, R., *Welfare Benefits* (Sweet & Maxwell, 1981).

Morgan, D., *Children in Care and Social Security* [1981] J.S.W.L. 196–214.

Ogus, A., and Barendt, E., *The Law of Social Security* (Butterworths, 1983).

Packman, J., *Child Care: Needs and Numbers* (Allen & Unwin, 1968).

Social Science Research and Intelligence Unit with Portsmouth Polytechnic, *Children on the Rates* (1980).

Tunnard, J., *Children in Care and Welfare Benefits* [1980] *Legal Action Group Bulletin 138.*
Wandsworth London Borough Council, *Charging for Social Services* (Wandsworth L.B.C., 1980).

Chapter 5

Bone, M., *Pre-school Children and the Need for Day Care* (DHSS, H.M.S.O., 1976).
Central Policy Review Staff, *Services for Young Children with Working Mothers* (H.M.S.O., 1978).
DHSS, *Intermediate Treatment—A Guide for the Regional Planning of New Forms of Treatment for Children in Trouble* (H.M.S.O., 1972).
DHSS, Local Authority Circular 77/1, *Children and Young Persons Act 1969—Intermediate Treatment* (1977).
DHSS, Local Authority Circular (83)6, *Criminal Justice Act 1982 Part I—Treatment of Young Offenders* (1983).
Dunlop, A., *Junior Attendance Centres*, Home Office Research Studies No. 60 (H.M.S.O., 1980).
Giller, H., and Morris, A., *Care and Discretion* (1981).
Hoggett, B., *Parents and Children* (Sweet & Maxwell, 1981).
Home Office, *Sentence of the Court* (H.M.S.O., 1978).
Home Office 1977—Home Office Circular 136/77 (C.S. 22/1977) *Attendance Centres* (1977).
Home Office Circular No. 42/1983, *Criminal Justice Act* (1982).
Home Office, App. C to Home Office Circular No. 135/1979, *Attendance Centres* (1979).
Jackson, B., and Jackson, S., *Childminder—A Study in Action Research* (Routledge and Kegan Paul, 1979).
Leeding, A., *Child Care Manual for Social Workers* (Butterworths, 1980).
McClintock, F. H., *Attendance Centres* (MacMillan, 1961).
McEwan, J. A., Commentaries on Cases at [1980] J.S.W.L. 48–52; and [1982] J.S.W.L. 172–175.
McEwan, J. A., *The Criminal Justice Act—Justice, Welfare or Confusion* [1983] M.L.R. 25.
Mayall, B., *Minder, Mother and Child* (University of London, Institute of Education, 1977).

Ministry of Health, *Nurseries and Childminders Regulation Act 1943* (as amended by section 60 of the Health Services and Public Health Act 1968)—Memorandum of Guidance for Local Health Authorities. Enclosure to Circular 36/68.

Ministry of Health, *Standards for the Day Care of Pre-school Children*—Memorandum of Guidance for Local Health Authorities. Enclosure to Circular 37/68.

Parker, H., Casburn, M., and Turnbull, D., *Receiving Juvenile Justice* (1981).

Plowden Report, The. *Children and their Primary Schools* (H.M.S.O., 1967).

Social Trends, 1981, Table 12 (H.M.S.O., 1981).

Stone, J., and Taylor, F., *The Parents Schoolbook* (Penguin, 1976).

Terry, J., "Childminding—A Time for Reform?" [1978–79] J.S.W.L. 389.

White Paper, *Young Offenders* Cmnd. 8045.

Chapter 6

Ball, A. G., "Why is Section 29 Misused?" [1967] *Brit. Hospital Journal* 1639.

Bean, P., *Compulsory Admissions to Mental Hospitals* (1980).

"The Mental Health Act 1959: Some Issues Concerning Rule Enforcement" (1975) 2 *Brit. J. of Law and Society* 225.

Butler Committee, *Report on Mentally Abnormal Offenders* Cmnd. 6244 (H.M.S.O., 1975).

Dawson, H. A. R., "Reasons for Compulsory Admission" in Wing, J. and Hailey, A., (eds.), *Evaluating a Community Psychiatric Service* (Oxford University Press, 1972).

DHSS, *Reform of Mental Health Legislation* Cmnd. 8405 (H.M.S.O., 1981).

DHSS, *A Review of the Mental Health Act 1959* (H.M.S.O., 1976).

DHSS, *A Review of the Mental Health Act 1959* Cmnd. 7320 (H.M.S.O., 1978).

Enoch, M. D., and Barker, J. C., "Misuse of Section 29: Fact or Fiction?" [1965] 3 *Lancet* 760.

Goffman, E., *Asylums* (Penguin, 1968).

Gostin, L., *A Human Condition* (MIND, 1975).

Gostin, L., "A Review of the Mental Health (Amendment) Act" (1982) 132 New L.J. 1127.

Gostin, L., "Contemporary Social Historical Perspectives on Mental Health Reform" (1983) 10 *Journal of Law and Society* 47.

Herbert, W. B., "The 'Urgent' Mental Patients" in *New Society*, February 2, 1965.

Hoggett, B., *Mental Health* (Sweet & Maxwell, 2nd ed., 1984).

Jones, K., *A History of the Mental Health Services* (R.K.P., 1972).

Percy Committee, *Report of Law Relating to Mental Illness and Mental Deficiency* Cmnd. 169 (H.M.S.O., 1957).

Szasz, T., *Ideology and Insanity* (Penguin, 1973).

Walker, N., and McCabe, S., *Crime and Insanity in England.*

Whitehead, A., "Patients' Rights and the Mental Health Act" in *World Medicine*, September 1974.

Chapter 7

C.O.H.S.E., *The Management of Violent or Potentially Violent Patients* (C.O.H.S.E., 1977).

Gostin, L., *A Human Condition* (MIND, 1975).

Gostin, L., "A Review of the Mental Health (Amendment) Act 1982" (1982) 132 New L.J. 1127.

Gostin, L., "Observations on Consent to Treatment and Review of Clinical Judgment in Psychiatry" (1981) 74 *Journal of Royal Society of Medicine* 742.

Gostin, L., *The Court of Protection: A Legal and Policy Analysis of the Guardianship of the Estate* (MIND, 1983).

Gostin, L., "The Merger of Incompetency and Certification" (1979) 2 *Int. J. of Law and Psychiatry* 127.

Heywood and Massey, *The Court of Protection* (Stevens, 1978).

Jacob, J., "The Right of the Mental Patient to His Psychosis" (1976) 38 M.L.R. 17.

Skegg, P., "A Justification for Medical Procedures Performed Without Consent" (1974) 90 L.Q.R. 512.

Szasz, T., "Lunatic Reform" in *Spectator*, December 4, 1982, p. 16.

Chapter 8

Carlin, J., *et al.*, "Civil Justice and the Poor" (1966) 1 *Law and Society Review* 9.
Gostin, L., *A Human Condition* (MIND, 1975).
Gostin, L., "Representing the Mentally Ill and Handicapped" *L.A.G. Bulletin* (1980).
Meacher, M., *New Methods of Mental Health Care* (Pergamon Press, 1979).

Chapter 9

de Smith, S., *Constitutional and Administrative Law* (Penguin, 1982).
DHSS, *Draft Guidelines for Approval of Social Workers* (DHSS, 1981).
Meacher, M., "Just Pretending?" (1983) 14 (No. 21) *Social Work Today* 11.
Seebohm Report, The. *Report of Committee on Local Authority and Allied Personal Social Services* Cmnd. 3703 (H.M.S.O., 1968).

Chapter 10

Ashworth, A., and Gostin, L., "The Mentally Disordered Offender & Sentencing Powers" [1984] C.L.R. 195.
Butler Committee, The. *Report on Mentally Abnormal Offenders* Cmnd. 6244 (H.M.S.O., 1975).
Gostin, L., *A Human Condition*, Vol. II. (MIND, 1977).
Gostin, L., Letter in *The Times*, January 28, 1982.
Hoggett, B., *Mental Health* (Sweet & Maxwell, 2nd ed., 1984).

Chapter 11

Age Concern, *The Attitudes of the Retired and Elderly* (Age Concern, 1974).

Brearley, P., *et al.*, *Admission to Residential Care* (Tavistock, 1980).

Brocklehurst, J. C., *et al.*, "Medical Screening of Old People accepted for Residential Care," *Lancet*, No. 8081, July 15, 1978.

Centre for Policy on Ageing, *Home Life: A Code of Practice for Residential Care* (London, 1984).

DHSS, "Some Aspects of Residential Care" (1976) 10 *Social Work Service* 3.

Goldberg, E. M., *et al.*, "Towards Accountability in Social Work: One Year's Intake to an Area Office" (1977) 7 *British Journal of Social Work* 257.

Grey, M., "Forcing Old People to leave their homes," *Community Care*, March 8, 1979, p. 19.

Morris, A., "The Disabled have their Act, Now they need the Action," *The Times*, May 26, 1982.

Wade, H. W., *Administrative Law* (Clarendon Press, 1982).

Index